FROM LATE ADOLESCENCE TO YOUNG ADULTHOOD

FROM LATE ADOLESCENCE TO YOUNG ADULTHOOD

By

David Dean Brockman, M.D.

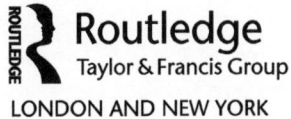

Routledge
Taylor & Francis Group

LONDON AND NEW YORK

First published 2003 by
Karnac Books Ltd

This edition published in 2011 by Karnac Books

Published 2018 by Routledge
2 Park Square, Milton Park, Abingdon, Oxon OX14 4RN
711 Third Avenue, New York, NY 10017, USA

Routledge is an imprint of the Taylor & Francis Group, an informa business

British Library Cataloguing in Publication Data
A C.I.P. for this book is available from the British Library

ISBN: 9781780490588 (pbk)

This book is dedicated to my late wife, Martha, whose unfailing support made this book possible; and our three children: Pamela, Sherrill, and David whose development into healthy, responsible, and productive young adults gave flesh and live feelings for this extraordinary period of life.

Table of Contents

Acknowledgments

Consolidation of the human personality occurs in a major way in late adolescence and young adulthood, making it a fascinating period of life that shows much promise for the future and for realizable ideals. These facts have been central to an interest of mine since I began psychoanalytic training in the early 1950s. My first training analyst, Dr. Harry B. Lee, stimulated and encouraged me with his skillful management of the transference, and especially his gift in dream interpretation, where I encountered some of the pertinent issues relevant to this period of development. I learned much from my second analyst, Dr. Thérèse Benedek, about narcissistic rage and the psychology of women. Since then, over the years those young persons I engaged in psychotherapy and psychoanalysis accelerated and expanded my understanding of late adolescence and young adulthood. New questions and problems were raised that required new solutions and/or resolution.

I am deeply indebted to all those young people as well as my colleagues, candidates I supervised at the Institute for Psychoanalysis, and psychiatric residents at the University of Illinois and Lutheran General Hospital in Park Ridge, Illinois, who shared their clinical case material with me in supervision and in clinical case conferences. Special mention in this regard is due Drs. Richard Baer, Bill Clark, David Edelstein, Martin Fine, Thomas Folsom, Richard Harris, Paul Hollinger, Mark

Levey, Fred Levin, Mel Prosen, and Marc Slutsky. They provided me with a wider and richer exposure to the psychodynamics of young adults than would otherwise have been possible. Their comments and understanding of their patients stimulated many hours of fruitful discussions that led to significantly greater insights.

Parts of the manuscript were read and constructively criticized by Drs. Morris Sklansky, Sol Altschul, Henry Seidenberg, George Moraitis, Charles Kligerman, Max Forman, Paul Tolpin, and Ernest Wolf. Their comments and suggestions were invaluable in improving the text conceptually and grammatically. Some parts of the manuscript were also read at the Institute's Wednesday Research meetings where lively discussions helped me to clarify my thinking and the written word. Dr. Richard Friedman offered many valuable suggestions regarding gender identity issues. A clearer understanding of homosexual orientation was made possible with the help and counsel of Drs. Bertram Cohler and Robert Galatzer-Levy as well as a number of gay male patients who sought analytic therapy for problems related to their sexual and gender issues.

Chapters 1 and 5 were previously published in earlier versions in the *Annual for Adolescent Psychiatry* and are reproduced here with the express permission of the editors of that publication for which I am grateful.

Dr. Arnold Goldberg encouraged me in my previous efforts in this area: *Late Adolescence: Psychoanalytic Studies*, published by International Universities Press, 1984. The present volume is a continuation of that stimulus and expanded conceptual themes expressed in the earlier work.

My daughter Pamela Brockman and her husband Pedro Jose Cevallos were very helpful in translating the Spanish references, particularly Maetzu's work on Don Juan, which the reknowned Ecuadoran scholar Gabriel Cevallos Garcia brought to my attention.

I am indebted to Mrs. Johanna Palmer Brockman for her assistance and encouragement in completing this project.

The editors of International Universities Press have been especially helpful at every step of the way, but I am especially appreciative of the numerous suggestions by Dr. Margaret Emery that immensely improved the text.

I wish to give special recognition to the incomparable assistance of the reference librarians at the University of Illinois Circle Library in locating reference materials and last but not least I want to thank Nancy Harvey and Bill Kelly at the Institute for Psychoanalysis Library for their expertise in obtaining some of the references.

Introduction

It is especially important at this time to study the personality growth of late adolescence into young adulthood since the median age of young people in the United States gradually increased from 27.9 years in 1970 and 30.0 years in 1980 to 30.6 years in 1982. This young adult age group under consideration here ranges from ages 20 to the early thirties. A person entering the adult world is considered by Levinson and his colleagues (Levinson, Darrow, Klein, Levinson, and McKee, 1978) to be 22 to 28 years of age, and the period of transition may be as long as five more years to age 33. Levinson et al. call the first part of this period of development a novice phase. "The primary overriding task of the novice phase is to make a place for oneself in the adult world and create a life structure that will be viable in the world and suitable for the self" (p. 72). However, young adulthood is frequently met with significant pathological regressions and failures in consolidation of the personality. Hanna Segal quotes Conrad's poignant personal description when he said the "green sickness of late youth descended on me and carried me off" (Segal, 1984, p. 5).

From 1972 to 1982, college enrollment increased by 35.3 percent representing about 3.2 million more students with 80 percent of the increase being women. Information on the current college population is somewhat sketchy since only the data from twenty-four states were reported in the *Statistical Abstracts*. The 1995 issue of the U.S. Department of Education *Digest of*

Education Statistics reports that college enrollment increased more slowly (about 30%), but there was an overall increase from 12.5 million to 14.3 million between 1983 and 1993 of whom 7.87 million were women and 6.42 million were men. The number of older students has been growing more rapidly than the number of younger students. "Between 1980 and 1990, the enrollment of students under age 25 increased by 3 percent. During the same period, enrollment of persons 25 and over rose by 34 percent. From 1990 to 2000, NCES projects a rise of 12 percent in enrollments of persons over 25 and an increase of 13 percent in the number under 25" (Table 169) (National Center for Education Statistics, *Digest of Education Statistics*, 1995, p. 167). In fact, only 20 percent of college students are younger than 22 (Zernike, 1999). Higgins (1988) quoted the College Board of Princeton, New Jersey, statistic that 46 percent of college students were 25 or older. The reason for this seems to be that undergraduate and graduate degrees are necessary requirements for employment and advancement in today's complex technological age.

The number of minority students rose from 15.7 percent in 1976 to 23.4 percent in 1993, due largely to Hispanic and Asian students, while the number of African-American students fluctuated between 1978 and 1993, eventually rising to 10.2 percent in 1993. Minority students were slightly more than 13 million, of whom 1.9 million were African Americans and nearly 1 million were Hispanics. This is an increase from slightly more than 10 million registered in state colleges and 3 million in private colleges reported just a few years ago. Black students attending the colleges supported by the United Negro College Fund increased in number by a record 20 percent from 1986 to 1991 representing over 50,000 new students (Jouzaitis, 1992). Thus, in just two years the number of college students increased by almost 700,000 despite the fact that government aid in the form of Pell grants and other types of loans had been sharply cut back. Between 1984 and 1985 and 1994 and 1995 costs at public colleges rose by 23 percent while costs at private institutions increased by 39 percent. In spite of this, most students do graduate. The national average of students graduating in four years from private colleges is 55 percent and 46 percent in public colleges. The remainder drop out for various reasons, not the least of which is the lack of sufficient funds. But more students are completing college. For example, "between 1982–83 and 1992–93, the number of associate, bachelor's, master's and doctor's degrees rose. Associate degrees increased 14 percent, bachelor's degrees increased 20 percent, master's degrees increased 27 percent, and doctor's degrees increased 29 percent during this period" (National Center for Educational Statistics, *Digest of Education Statistics,* 1995, p. 168).

Increasing opportunities for women in areas including business, accounts for the fact that women receiving bachelor's degrees increased by 29 percent between 1982 and 1983 and 1992 and 1993, while the increase for men was 11 percent. Also, almost as many women as men are now enrolled in business and professional schools. It seems too that graduate degrees are becoming almost as necessary to secure employment as undergraduate degrees were in the past. In some medical schools, there are now more women enrolled than men. The same is true for American veterinary medical colleges where two-thirds of students are women and nearly one-third of veterinarians are women (Wukas, 1997).

Sexual behavior of the 18 to 29 age group is surprisingly conventional, according to the survey by Michael, Gagnon, Laumann, and Kolata (1994). Sixty-four percent of men and 66 percent of women respectively report a frequency of sex of two to three times per week. Over half of the women and three-quarters of men were either cohabiting or were married. These figures conclusively point to a more conventional pattern than existed a decade or more earlier when promiscuity and multiple partners were thought to be more common. The inference here is that the AIDS crisis has made couples more cautious in their sexual behavior. Sax, Astin, Korn, and Mahoney (1996) report a nationwide study that fewer students (41%) engage in casual sex than in previous years and larger numbers (72%) prefer volunteer community service to political activities.

This study of the young adult takes up where the *Late Adolescence: Psychoanalytic Studies* (Brockman, 1984) book left off, but the present work is not merely a simple continuation of the concepts and developmental issues raised by the previous contribution. Conceptualizations of late adolescence are expanded upon and applied to the young adult population. Adulthood is defined here by the sociologist Garbarino (1978) as an operational concept involving those qualities of human development that lead to competence and accountability in a variety of areas so that "an individual is prepared to be held legally and socially responsible for himself and others" (p. 170). In a more specific sense, this book contains a consideration of the very complex issues of achieving socialization into young adulthood: identity formation, intimacy, career choice, and internalization of those values and goals which together with gender and sexual identities are consolidated in the personality and are regarded as the central qualities and tasks of the young adult. Also, the biopsychosocial systems model followed here, which was originally proposed by Engel (1977, 1980), is a method of organizing and structuring the multiplicity of data collected about individuals healthy or otherwise. Schwartz and Wiggins (1986) further clarify the role of meaning in organizing and regulating experience and behavior in human systems. Meanings are assimilated through both development and socialization modalities and may reduce some aspects of complexity in the interaction between biological and psychosocial systems.

Homosexual men seem to consolidate their sexual preferences during this period of life (19.3 years, according to Dank,
1971; Friedman, 1988) while homosexual women consolidate
their sexual identities two or three years later than men. Also,
changes in societal acceptance of gay lifestyles along with certain legal and social services have made it easier for gays to
"come out." Some gay adolescents may declare their sexual
preferences in high school. There is a public magnet high
school in New York City where gay students can study without
harassment from other students. Some homosexual men report erotic arousal much earlier (ages 4–13) and not necessarily stimulated by contact with known homosexuals. Further,
they report that they experience themselves as different from
other boys since they don't like rough-and-tumble sports and
consider themselves as having been effeminate (Friedman,
1988, p. 175). Boxer's study (1990) of homosexuality in adolescence includes reports of same-sex fantasies about the same
age in both boys and girls (between 11 and 12). However, the
key word here is *consolidation* of the personality, and that process is usually not completed in most people until young adulthood and sometimes much later.

Siegel (1988) follows Socarides' (1988; Socarides and Volkan, 1991) psychopathological views about the development of
a gay lifestyle in women, including the dynamics of a pregenital, preverbal nonawareness of a vagina and a failure to engage
in age-appropriate play. She attributes special meaning to early
preoedipal castration anxiety. Freud's caution in his paper on
a case of female homosexuality (1920) is still cogent today to
the effect that "it is not for psychoanalysis to solve the problem
of homosexuality. It must rest content with disclosing the psychical mechanisms that resulted in determining the object
choice, and with tracing back the paths from them to the instinctual dispositions" (p. 171).

Boxer, Cohler, Herdt, and Irwin (1993) cite the lack of prospective longitudinal developmental studies as contrasted to the previous predominately retrospective studies. They especially decry the serious limitations of retrospective research following Sigmund Freud's similar warnings concerning retrospective linear assumptions about development with such a great emphasis on childhood experiences (1920, p. 167) without considering other factors. Furthermore, false conclusions can be drawn from people who seek help from mental health care workers for distress about their sexual orientation, if they are based only on those retrospective linear assumptions. Longitudinal life course studies are critical for the acquisition of solid data about the development of gay and lesbian youth and a "developmental perspective can be a useful framework from which to examine the effects and interrelation of historical time and sociocultural contexts on individual development" (p. 272). They say such newer research strategies of quantitative and qualitative measurements would be an improvement over cross-sectional and retrospective studies of the remembered past that tend to ignore discontinuities in development of individuals as well as across groups. Postponement of marriage due to lengthy postgraduate educational programs leads to serious psychological problems, not the least of which is a delay in finding a suitable mate. In already existing marriages, prolonged educational programs such as those for medical residencies, create serious marital discord (Gabbard and Menninger, 1989). Of the 320 couples studied, 93 percent of the male spouses with an average age of 44.6 years were somewhat older than the young adult population. Younger groups would most certainly reveal the same data, however, and members of this older group were still struggling with the same issues that are common to the younger group because prolonged educational programs delay emotional and social development in this older group. Levinson (1967) considered socialization processes and socialization theory regarding medical students. The implication of his study is that the pressures of medical school seriously influence socialization and developmental processes. Specifically, in the Gabbard and Menninger (1989) study, emotional intimacy was severely limited and closeness produced much discomfort and discord in the marital relationships. The character structure of the physicians studied was of the compulsive type accompanied by much "self-doubt, guilt feelings, and exaggerated sense of responsibility, reluctance to take vacations from work, difficulty setting limits, and chronic feelings of 'not doing enough' " (p. 2379).

The physical health of young adults is usually and generally quite good, but this population is at the highest risk for the onset of serious headache syndrome. An epidemiological study (Linet, Stewart, Celentano, Zeigler, and Sprecher, 1989) found the prevalence of headache to be 6.1 percent in males and 14.0 percent in females ages 12 to 29 in the young adult population studied in a rural county in Maryland. A study of Israeli adolescents (Nathan, Frenkel, and Kugelmass, 1994) growing up into young adulthood revealed that those raised in a kibbutz were more likely to suffer a major depression than those raised in an urban household. Nathan et al. cite as a reason for this the kibbutzniks having been deprived of maternal care giving during the critical period of development in early childhood. Goodman (1999) found a close correlation between suicide among late adolescents and young adults and low family income levels. Increased risk for suicide in homosexual and lesbian young adult populations is not necessarily due to substance abuse or other psychiatric comorbity problems (Herrell et al., 1999), and in a longitudinal study from birth to 21 years of age by Ferguson, Horwood, and Beautrais (1999) confirmed an increase of suicidality in gay and lesbian young adults. Further, Friedman (1999) calls for more research in this area to supplement these findings, especially in terms of the immunodeficiency virus status of this group. In a study of seventy-two gay, lesbian, and bisexual youths by Floyd, Stein, Harter, Allison, and Nye (1999) separation-individuation proceeded normally when individuals were accepting of their sexual orientation identity.

Identity (Erikson, 1956, 1966; Marcia, 1980) is seen to arise in a complex interaction of social and psychological learning experiences between the individual and his or her environment, with internalization of qualities and characteristics from identification processes. Parallel to and concomitant with internalization processes are socialization processes that intermingle to account for the extraordinarily complex and intricate developmental achievements during this period of life. Age stratification lays an important role in the socialization process too (Riley, Johnson, and Foner, 1972). Socialization of young people "implies the uneventful acquisition of increasingly adult-like beliefs" (Olmsted and Smith, 1980, p. 182). It is here that the concepts of socialization raised by Vygotsky (1960; cited in Wertsch, 1985) and others (Neugarten and Datan, 1973; Looft, 1973; Ahamma, 1973) are pertinent and most fruitful to our understanding of the late adolescent and young adult who experiences a major expansion of his cognitive and linguistic skills in the context of educational and other socialization experiences associated with an educational environment. Linguistic skills are enhanced, Vygotsky claims (cited in Wertsch, 1985), through the mediation of semiotics, that is, various signs and symbols. An increasingly complex language capacity for formal operations and for communication is central to Vygotsky's theory (1934). Educational experiences, for Vygotsky, are the most important medium for facilitating and internalizing what the social and cultural milieu has to offer to an already existing internal genetic and constitutional milieu. Significant internal structure of the mind is thus added. It is relatively easy to use the theory to make the connection between social, psychological, and constitutional contributions to the development of mind. Durkheim (1911) agrees for an even earlier stage of development by stating that: "Education is the influence exercised by the adult generations on those that are not yet ready for social life. Its object is to arouse and to develop in the child [and young adults] a certain number of physical, intellectual and moral states which are demanded of him by both the political society as a whole and the special milieu for which he is specially destined" (p. 71).

Zuschlag and Whitbourne (1994) studied over 300 college students at the University of Rochester. They learned that college seniors from the 1960s, 1970s, and 1980s consistently had higher psychosocial developmental scores than sophomores and juniors. Specifically, they were higher on measurements of Erikson's psychosocial stages. Also, women seniors were generally more mature than male seniors. Obviously, the senior year of college coincides with a consolidation process that was demonstrated by Zuschlag and Witbourne's study. Even earlier, Olmsted and Smith (1980) have demonstrated that high-school seniors "acquire more commonsense views of social life that come increasingly to resemble those of adults in their communities" (p. 181). What they studied were high school students' conceptions of mental health. Zern (1985) showed that while college students saw authorities as more important earlier in life, the individual became more important to them later on. Macooby (1984) has decried the fact that research in child development has pursued two divergent paths: cognitive and social–emotional, without much integration. Macooby's "objective is to consider the way we have thought about socialization within the family and to ask in what way age-linked developmental change may be implicated in socialization" (p. 318). He argues that neither "traditional unidirectional models nor the more recent interactive ones, are developmental in the strong sense of that word" (p. 318). In the traditional model of child developmental studies, researchers are looking for different patterns of parental behavior that are associated with differences among children. He then claims it is no longer wise to consider socialization as unidirectional but rather as interactional and dyadic. Both parents influence the child differently when both are present together than when either one is alone with the child (Steinberg, 1987). Siblings also play an important role. But socialization research has not been able as yet to throw much light on the role of gender related behavior in longitudinal processes, particularly in determining the child's goals, plans, or instrumental behavior. The child soon enough increasingly resists the intrusion of parental influences and sets his own "gyroscope" (Ginott, 1965).

However much the educational process aids in the socialization process, there are now increasing demands on the late adolescent in transition to young adulthood resulting from rapid and massive changes in the socioeconomic system. Conflicting ideologies, and a multitude of demographic changes such as divorce, desertion of families by fathers, drug-related crime, and increasing prison populations, also have a major impact. Racially segregated ghettos, neglect and abuse of children, and drive-by shootings, all produce gross challenges to and resultant failures in the acquisition of socially acceptable standards of adult behavior. Moreover, the culture in the United States has become more pluralistic and more complex in recent years so that the requirements for adulthood have become more complex than they were in the 1980s. Political socialization studies such as that of Rogers and Tedin (1976) suggest that children and adolescents acquire political views earlier than was previously thought, and their views persist on into adulthood. They quote a study by R. Jones (1976) to the effect that is even more true today that the racial composition of the classroom, teacher attitudes, and the legal atmosphere of the school situation make the school system "a community force" (p. 294) with the result that students become more political, especially when there are open, participatory classrooms where controversial opinions are expressed (Travers, 1983).

Cognitive development in the young adult proceeds from formal operations in adolescence, to postformal thought processes in young adulthood, and the development of higher moral and ethical values later on in young adulthood (Commons, Richards, and Armon, 1984). At "around the age of 18 or 19 people start to be able to coordinate several aspects of two or more abstractions in *Level 9 abstract systems*" (Fischer, Hand, and Russell, 1984). Then around age 25, "individuals can begin to integrate abstract systems to form *Level 10 general principles . . .*" (p. 52), including systematic and metasystematic reasoning (Richards and Commons, 1984, p. 96). Basseches (1984) uses a different term, *dialectal thinking*, to emphasize the "constitutive and interactive relationships through which systems evolve and change" (p. 236). Arlin (1984) suggests the presence of a relativistic logical system of thought in young adults that is either manifested in contractions or expansions in the service of "problem solving, decision making and the discovery-oriented behaviors of scientists" (p. 263). Problem finding is also present as an effort to fill gaps in knowledge and similarly raise pertinent questions about previously unanswered and disregarded issues. Sinnott (1984) extends this concept of relativistic thinking into solving problems in the area of interpersonal relationships. Postconventional reasoning, furthermore, contains development and adoption of higher moral and ethical standards and values (Armon, 1984).

Identity (Erikson, 1956, 1966; R. Grinberg, 1966; L. Grinberg and R. Grinberg, 1974; Abend, 1974; Holland, 1985) involves vocational career choice but also involves organized and enduring characterological and affective states such as the grouchy, depressed loner; the cheerful, optimistic gregarious person; or the angry, hostile, mean person. The misogynist, the misanthrope, the curmudgeon, or the maven are familiar to everyone as well as the imposter, the conman, the moocher, the trickster, the hero, or the jock. Identity could refer to the college one graduates from or a regional or national geographic location or a political, religious, ethnic, or economic status (Pollock, 1983). Identity can be seen as an ego function or a self structure as well as a constitutional state such as Osler's general classifications of the "lark" versus the "owl" personality types. My definition of identity is a synthesis of different accretions in the personality in the light of significant internalization and socialization processes which merge to form the multifaceted biopsychosocial identity of any given individual. Also, infant observational studies must be integrated with clinical psychoanalytic data (Stern, 1977, 1985; Emde, 1983, 1985, 1988; Sorce and Emde, 1981; Speers, McFarland, Arnaud, and Curry, 1971; Shapiro and Emde, 1992; Wolff, 1996). A capacity for intimacy is considered to be the result of a strong identity formation and the establishment of fidelity to a love object. The *Journal of Adolescence* (1996) was devoted to more current conceptualizations of identity development encompassing social, historical, ethnic, environmental, and contextual issues that emphasize identity as an adaptational process. R. Grinberg (1966) and R. Grinberg and L. Grinberg (1971, 1974) spell out the processes of identity formation through the analytic process with analysands while Joseph and Widlocher (1983) defined identity formation in the psychoanalyst.

Gender and sexual identity are considered from biological and psychological perspectives. Gender identity is differentiated from sexual identity in that the gender identity of a person is constituted from those unique masculine or feminine qualities in a personality, while sexual identity is composed of biological and physiological factors. Clinical examples are given to illustrate these differences.

The chapter on Don Juan takes up the classical character in Fra Tirso de Molina's original play (1630). There have been many versions of the play over the ages, the best known being da Ponte's libretto for Mozart's opera *Don Giovanni*. The single case study method (Stephenson, 1953; Jones and Windholz, 1990) is employed here to amplify and clarify the thesis raised by the literary character that Don Juan is pursuing the idealized woman who represents the primary attachment to an idealized mother. Narcissistic rage (Kohut, 1971) is taken up in connection with Akhilleus in Homer's *The Iliad* (Lattimore, 1951) who withdrew from battle after he was publicly and sorely humiliated by Agamemnon who had taken Briseis, the beautiful woman who was Akhilleus's prize. Akhilleus sulked and brooded in his tent and then entered into a deeper melancholic state when his alter ego, Patroklos, was killed in battle. Akhilleus recovered first after undergoing a mourning process and second after undergoing a rapprochement with Priam, the father of several men and boys Akhilleus had killed in revenge for the death of Patroklos. Clinical material is used to buttress the thesis that narcissistic rage is derived from a series of childhood humiliations. The case material reported in the Don Juan and Akhilleus chapters is limited to certain specific characteristics and dynamics that remind one of the literary characters. For example, The "Don Juan" patient was constantly seeking out the idealized mother in the transference to merge with her in order to complete an uncompleted self, while the "Akhilleus" patient's alter ego relationship with me in the transference assisted him in mourning and constructing a solid self structure.

The motives for achieving power over others are taken up in chapter 6. It appears that the author of *The Prince* (Machiavelli, 1532) has been misrepresented in modern times in that he is now popularly seen as evil and calculating, but if taken in the context of his times he was simply advising a political leader on how to remain in power. There is some evidence to indicate he was really a true republican in the generic sense of the term, and philosophically a supporter of popular government. A clinical example is given to illustrate and expand on some of the ideas gathered from the literature.

Creativity in young adults is generated when there is a close special relationship with another person or persons in reality or in fantasy. This thesis is documented in a number of instances of genius over the course of history. Mathematical geniuses seem to be able to create in the absence of a significant relationship, but the subject matter is naturally very abstract, and mathematical geniuses notoriously live rather isolated and asocial lives. They are often difficult to get along with socially, and they have a love affair with abstractions and numbers. Newton is frequently cited as one of the more notorious examples of someone who led a socially isolated life, but at the same time one could cite other creative mathematicians who successfully negotiate relationships with others. The thesis espoused here, though, deserves serious consideration since there are many creative people whose lives demonstrate that their creativity originates within a close relationship with a significant self–self-object relationship. Oremland's (1997) masterful synthesis of the psychoanalytic theory of creativity specifies an internal object relationship that is critically important in creative individuals. In the light of this concept Newton's intense relationship with his mother over a long period of time would be consistent with the thesis presented here.

The concluding chapter summarizes the phase-specific developmental tasks of the young adult. Passage into young adulthood is clearly not easy and is made more difficult and complicated because options and opportunities for career choice are more numerous today than ever before. Specific intellectual skills are engaged by the largely fortuitous impact of teachers in high school and college on the late adolescent and young adult, resulting in a narrowing of interests and limitation of opportunities. Socialization processes and social learning in earlier phases influence learning to adapt and cope with later social learning (Cavins and Hood, 1983). Also, finding a suitable love object is more difficult when the young adult leaves the school setting and returns home to live for economic or other reasons after graduating from college, where greater independence and autonomy are enjoyed. This book brings together some of the contributions from the disciplines of developmental psychology, sociology, infant research, and research in psychoanalysis (Luborsky and Crits-Christof, 1990) as they apply to the psychology of young adults.

REFERENCES

Abend, S. (1974), Problems of identity, theoretical and clinical applications. *Psychoanal. Quart.*, 43:606–637.

Ahamma, I. M. (1973), Social-learning theory as a framework for the study of adult personality development. In: *Life-Span Developmental Psychology*, ed. P. B. Baltes & K. W. Schaie. New York: Academic Press, pp. 253–284.

Arlin, P. A. (1984), Adolescent and adult thought: A structural interpretation. In: *Beyond Formal Operations*, ed. M. L. Commons, F. A. Richards, & C. Armon. New York: Praeger, pp. 258–271.

Armon, S. (1984), Ideal of the good life and moral judgement: Ethical reasoning across the lifespan. In: *Beyond Formal Operations*, ed. M. L. Commons, F. A. Richards, & S. Armon. New York: Praeger, pp. 357–380.

Basseches, M. (1984), Dialectal thinking as a metasystematic form of cognitive organization. In: *Beyond Formal Operations*, ed. M. L. Commons, F. A. Richards, & S. Armon. New York: Praeger, pp. 216–238.

Boxer, A. M. (1990), *Life Course Transitions of Gay and Lesbian Youth's Sexual Identity, Development, and Parent-Child Relationships*. Unpublished doctoral dissertation. Committee on Human Development. The University of Chicago.

———— Cohler, B. J., Herdt, G., & Irwin, F. (1993), The study of gay and lesbian teenagers: Life course, "coming out" and well being. In: *Handbook of Clinical Research and Practice with Adolescents*, ed. P. H. Tolan & B. J. Cohler. New York: John Wiley, pp. 249–280.

Brockman, D. D. (1984), *Late Adolescence: Psychoanalytic Studies*. New York: International Universities Press.

Cavins, R. B., & Hood, K. E. (1983), Continuity in social development: A comparative perspective in individual difference prediction. In: *Life-Span Development and Behavior*, ed. P. B. Baltes & O. G. Brim, Jr. New York: Academic Press, pp. 301–358.

Commons, M. L., Richards, F. A., & Armon, S., Eds. (1984), *Beyond Formal Operations*. New York: Praeger.

Dank, B. (1971), Coming out in the gay world. *Psychiatry*, 4:184–197.

Durkheim, E. (1911), *Education and Sociology*, tr. S. D. Fox. New York: Free Press, 1956.

———— (1980), The clinical application of the biopsychosocial model. *Amer. J. Psychiatry*, 137:535–544.

Emde, R. (1983), The prerepresentational self and its affective core. *The Psychoanalytic Study of the Child*, 38:165–192. New Haven, CT: Yale University Press.

———— (1985), Emotional availability, shared meaning, and the origins of "We-Go." Presentation at the Chicago Psychoanalytic Society, June 25.

———— (1988), Development terminable and interminable: Innate motivational factors from infancy. *Internat. J. Psycho-Anal.*, 69:23–42.

Engel, G. L. (1977), The need for a new medical model: A challenge for biomedicine. *Science*, 196:129–136.

Erikson, E. H. (1956), The problem of ego identity. *J. Amer. Psychanal. Assn.*, 4:56–121.

———— (1966), Ontogeny of ritualization. In: *Psychoanalysis—A General Psychology*, ed. R. M. Loewenstein, L. M. Newman, M. Schur, & A. L. Solnit. New York: International Universities Press, pp. 601–621.

———— (1977), *Toys and Reasons. In: Stages in Ritualization Experience*. New York: W. W. Norton.

Ferguson, D. M., Horwood, L. J., & Beautrais, A. L. (1999), Is sexual orientation related to mental health problems and suicidality in young people? *Arch. Gen. Psych.*, 56:876–880.

Fischer, K. W., Hand, H. H., & Russell, S. (1984), The development of abstractions in adolescence and adulthood. In: *Beyond Formal Operations*, ed. M. L. Commons, F. A. Richards, & S. Armon. New York: Praeger, pp. 43–73.

Floyd, F. J., Stein, T. S., Harter, K. S. M., Allison, A., & Nye, C. L. (1999), Gay, lesbian, and bisexual youths: Separation-individuation, parental attitudes, identity consolidation, and well-being. *J. Youth & Adol.*, 28:719–739.

Freud, S. (1920), The psychogenesis of a case of homosexuality in a woman. *Standard Edition*, 18:145–172. London: Hogarth Press, 1955.

Friedman, R. C. (1988), *Male Homosexuality*. New Haven, CT: Yale University Press.

———— (1999), Commentary. *Arch. Gen. Psych.*, 56:887–888.

Gabbard, G., & Menninger, R. (1989), The psychology of postponement in the medical marriage. *J. Amer. Med. Assn.*, 16:261:2378–2381.

Garbarino, J. (1978), *The role of schools in socialization to adulthood. The Educational Forum*, 42:169–181.

Ginott, H. G. (1965), *Between Parent and Child*. New York: Macmillan.

Goodman, E. (1999), The role of socioeconomic status gradients in explaining differences in U.S. adolescents' health. *Amer. J. Public Health.* 89:1522–1528.

Grinberg, L., & Grinberg, R. (1971), *Identidad y Cambio*. Buenos Aires: Kargieman.

——— ——— (1974), The problem of identity and the psychoanalytical process. *Internat. Rev. Psychoanal.*, 1:499–507.

Grinberg, R. (1966), The acquisition of the sense of identity in the psychoanalytic process, tr. P. Brockman. *Rev. Psychoanal.*, 8:247–254 (Uruguay).

Herrell, R., Goldberg, J., True, W. R., Ramakrishnau, V., Lyons, M., Eisen, S., & Tsuang, M. T. (1999), Sexual orientation and suicidality. *Arch. Gen. Psych.*, 56:867–874.

Higgins, R. (1988), The new college kid might not be a kid at all. *Chicago Tribune*, April 10, Sect. 5, p. 4.

Holland, N. (1985), *The I*. New Haven, CT: Yale University Press.

Jones, E. E., & Windholz, M. (1990), The psychoanalytic case study: Toward a method for systematic inquiry. *J. Amer. Psychoanal. Assn.*, 38:985–1015.

Jones, R. (1976), Institutional change and socialization research. *Youth & Society*, 8:277–298.

Joseph, E. D., & Widlocher, D. (1983), *The Identity of the Psychoanalyst*, IPA Monograph No. 2. New York: International Universities Press.

Jouzaitis, C. (1992), Black colleges get bigger and better. *Chicago Tribune*, June 7, Sect. 1, p. 1.

Kohut, H. (1971), *The Analysis of the Self*. New York: International Universities Press.

Lattimore, R. (1951), *The Iliad of Homer*. Chicago: University of Chicago Press.

Levinson, D., Darrow, C., Klein, E., Levinson, M., & McKee, B. (1978), *The Seasons of a Man's Life*. New York: Ballantine.

Levinson, D. J. (1967), Medical education and the theory of adult socialization. *Med. Edu. & Social.*, 84:253–265.

Linet, M. S., Stewart, W. F., Celentano, D. D., Zeigler, D., & Sprecher, M. (1989), An epidemiologic study of headache among adolescents and young adults. *J. Amer. Med. Assn.*, 15:2211–2216.

Looft, W. R. (1973), Socialization and personality throughout the life span: An examination of contemporary psychological approaches. In: *Lifespan Developmental Psychology*, ed. P. B. Baltes & K. W. Schaie. New York: Analytic Press, pp. 25–52.

Luborsky, L., & Crits-Christoph, P. (1990), *Understanding Transference: The CCRT Method*. New York: Basic Books.

Machiavelli, N. (1532), *The Prince*, ed. & tr. Q. Skinner & R. Price. Cambridge, U.K.: Cambridge University Press, 1988.

Macooby, E. E. (1984), Socialization and developmental change. *Child Develop.* 55:317–328.

Marcia, J. E. (1980), Identity in adolescence. In: *Handbook of Adolescent Psychology*, ed. J. Adelson. New York: John Wiley, pp. 159–187.

Michael, R. T., Gagnon, J. H., Laumann, E. O., & Kolata, G. (1994), *Sex in America*. New York: Little, Brown.

de Molina, T. (1630), Don Juan. In: *Great Spanish Plays in English Translation*, ed. A. Flores. New York: Dover, 1991, pp. 81–133.

Nathan, M., Frenkel, E., & Kugelmass, S. (1994), From adolescence to adulthood: Development of psychopathology in kibbutz and town subjects. *J. Youth & Adol.*, 22:605–621.

National Center for Education Statistics (1995), *Digest of Education Statistics*. Washington, DC: National Center for Education Statistics, U.S. Department of Education.

Neugarten, B., & Datan, N. (1973), Sociological perspectives on the life cycle. In: *Lifespan Developmental Psychology*, ed. P. B. Baltes & K. W. Schaie. New York: Academic Press, pp. 53–69.

Olmsted, D. W., & Smith, D. L. (1980), The socialization of youth into the American mental health belief system. *J. Health & Soc. Behav.*, 21:181–194.

Oremland, J. D. (1997), *The Origins and Psychodynamics of Creativity*. Madison, CT: International Universities Press.

Pollock, G. H. (1983), Self and identity: The psychoanalyst, psychoanalysis, and society. In: *The Identity of the Psychoanalyst*, ed. E. D. Joseph & D. Widlocher. IPA Monograph No. 2. New York: International Universities Press, pp. 195–206.

Richards, F. A., & Commons, M. L. (1984), Systematic, metasystematic, and cross-paradigmatic reasoning: A case for stages of reasoning beyond formal reasoning. In: *Beyond Formal Operations*, ed. M. L. Commons, F. A. Richards, & S. Armon. New York: Praeger, pp. 92–119.

Riley, M. W., Johnson, M., & Foner, A., Eds. (1972), *Ageing and Society*. New York: Rusell Sage Foundation.

Rogers, H. R., & Tedin, K. L. (1976), Political socialization: Assessment of theoretical approaches, methods and findings. 1. Introduction. *Youth & Soc.*, 8:101–116.

Sax, L., Astin, A. W., Korn, W. S., & Mahoney, K. M. (1996), *The American Freshman: National Norms For Fall 1996*. Los Angeles, CA. Higher Education Research Institute, University of California at Los Angeles.

Schwartz, M. A., & Wiggins, O. P. (1986), Systems and the structuring of meaning: Contributions to a biopsychosocial medicine. *Amer. J. Psychiatry*, 143:1213–1221.

Segal, H. (1984), Joseph Conrad and the mid-life crisis. *Internat. Rev. Psychoanal.*, 11:3–10.

Shapiro, T., & Emde, R. N. (1992), Affect: Developmental perspectives, introduction. *J. Amer. Psychoanal. Assn.*, 39:5–34.

Siegel, E. (1988), *Female Homosexuality*. Hillsdale, NJ: Analytic Press.

Sinnott, J. D. (1984), Postformal reasoning: The relativistic stage. In: *Beyond Formal Operations*, ed. M. L. Commons, F. A. Richards, & S. Armon. New York: Praeger, pp. 298–325.

Socarides, C. (1988), *The Preoedipal Origin and Psychoanalytic Therapy of Sexual Perversions*. Madison, CT: International Universities Press.

——— Volkan, V., Eds. (1991), *The Homosexualities and The Therapeutic Process*. Madison, CT: International Universities Press.

Sorce, J. F., & Emde, R. N. (1981), Mother's presence is not enough. *Develop. Psychol.*, 17:737–745.

Speers, R. W., McFarland, M. B., Arnaud, S. H., & Curry, N. E. (1971), Recapitulation of separation–individuation processes when the normal three-year-old enters nursery school. In: *Separation-Individuation*, ed. J. M. McDevitt & C. Settlage. New York: International Universities Press, pp. 297–321.

Steinberg, L. (1987), Sex differences in family relations at adolescence. Special issue. *J. Youth & Adol.*, 16:191–312.

Stephenson, W. (1953), *The Study of Behavior: Q-Technique and Its Methodology*. Chicago: University of Chicago Press.

Stern, D. N. (1977), *The First Relationship*. Cambridge, MA: Harvard University Press.

——— (1985), *The Interpersonal World of the Infant*. New York: Basic Books.

Travers, E. F. (1983), The role of schools in political socialization reconsidered. Evidence from 1970–1979. *Youth & Soc.*, 14:475–500.

Vygogtsky, L. S. (1934), *Thinking and Speech: Psychological Investigations*. Moscow: Gosudarstvennoe Sotsial'np Ekonomicheskoe Izdatel'stvo.

——— (1960), *The Development of Higher Mental Functions*. Moscow: Izadetel'stvo Akademii Pedagoficheskikh Nauk.

Wertsch, J. V. (1985), *Vygotsky and the Social Formation of Mind*. Cambridge, MA: Harvard University Press.

Wolff, P. H. (1996), The irrelevance of infant observations for psychoanalysis. *J. Amer. Psychoanal. Assn.*, 44:369–392.

Wukas, M. (1997), More veterinarians are women. *Chicago Tribune*, Feb. 2, Sect. 13, p. 3.

Zern, D. S. (1985), The expressed preference of different ages of adolescents for assistance in the development of moral values. *Adol.*, 20:405–423.

Zernike, K. (1999), Ageing student body. *Chicago Tribune*, Nov. 7, Section 13, p. 8.

Zuschlag, M. K., & Whitbourne, S. K. (1994), Psychosocial development in three generations of college students. *J. Youth & Adol.*, 23:567–575.

Chapter 1

The Psychoanalytic Assessment of Young Adults

Psychoanalytic assessment of the personalities of young adults implies the study of certain intrapsychic states which are taken up in this chapter in terms of clinical and developmental issues (Rapaport and Gill, 1959). Assessment of young adults by the psychoanalytic method must, first of all, take into account how well any individual has succeeded in negotiating and working through the phase-specific tasks and conflicts associated with late adolescence (Spiegel, 1961; Adatto, 1980), and by inference all previous phases of development (Blos, 1962). Transition from late adolescence to young adulthood (Eisenstadt, 1956; Block with N. Haan, 1971; Vaillant, 1977; Levinson, Arrow, Klein, Levinson, and McGee, 1978; Arnstein, 1989) may be a relatively continuous, unconflicted growth process (Offer and Offer, 1975), or mark identity achievement status (Marcia, 1980; Holland, 1985; Josselson, 1989). My clinical experience with late adolescents and young adults suggests that most, if not all, are concerned with phase specific tasks, which often become involved in conflict that in turn produces clinically observable symptoms. It is true my clinical observations are

An earlier version of this chapter was published in *Adolescent Psychiatry*, (1989) Vol. 16, pp. 246–258. Permission granted for reprinting by the author and the Editor of *Adolescent Psychiatry*.

1

derived from a skewed patient population, but my observation of nonpatient populations (including my children, those of my colleagues, and close friends) is that similar issues arise in nonclinical instances with more or less frequent if transient symptom formation.

Those individuals without serious symptomatology obviously do not seek therapy and work out their issues more or less independently or else maintain a relatively uneasy equilibrium.

Clinical vignettes are included, where appropriate, to amplify the concepts related to the young adult. In order to proceed in an orderly way to outline and fill out a credible psychoanalytic assessment of young men and women, I shall survey some of those areas of personality functioning that are important for understanding this developmental phase. This is the period of life following college for some, graduate school for others, and for those entering the job market directly out of high school. It is the time for marriage and starting a family, for entering a profession, building a career, and a "settling down" into recognizable patterns of behavior. All these developments are a result of the successful integration or resolution of the tasks of the adolescent phase, especially the late adolescent phase.

Early on, Fountain (1961) singled out five qualities of college students that undergo change as they mature: intensity and volatility of emotion, need for immediate gratification, ineffective reality testing, failures in self-criticism, and an egocentric view of the world. These qualities change at different rates, but as Fountain points out, in general, egocentrism gives way to a more global view of the world, and the young adult relates to other people as having rights and privileges distinct from his or her own. Emotions are more modulated and are put into the service of enhancing relationships. Normally, the adolescent personality as it traverses into young adulthood undergoes a consolidation process, and part of that process is characterized by certain transitional phenomena (Connell and Furman, 1984). These transitional phenomena may consist of manifest or latent variables that are specific for late adolescence: (1) adult sexual object choice; (2) consolidation of sexual and gender identities; (3) expansion of ego functions which become less concerned with conflict (Hartmann, 1950, 1952, 1955, 1958) resulting in: (4) the freeing up of energies for creative and productive work in a chosen vocation; (5) the development of more intimate object relations and less involvement with narcissistic relations with others, peers as well as younger and older persons; (6) significant restructuring of the superego and ego ideal (Hartmann and Loewenstein, 1962; Jacobson, 1964; Kernberg, 1975, 1987; Chused, 1987a,b, 1988); (7) a firm harmonious consolidation of the structures that will compose the young adult personality or character; and (8) preparations for parenthood (Benedek, 1959, 1970). Some of these structures, for purposes of elaboration, are considered to be enhanced versions or transformations of previously formed and enduring or stable aspects of personality functioning. One must always remember that in any young adult there are unresolved residues or fixations from previous developmental phases, and the potential for regressive response to developmental crises must be assessed. Newly formed structures appear at this time as progressive contributions to the young adult's character, but are often the most vulnerable to regressive change. The young adult's idealization of the analyst contributes to developmental progression as a transitional phenomenon (Chused, 1987b). Wolf, Gedo, and Terman (1972), from a self psychological standpoint, viewed the transformation of the self as *the* major task of adolescence. One of the dangers encountered at this time is an increased vulnerability of and failures in cohesion of the self when parental selfobjects are deidealized. Wolf (1982) has observed this task to be a continuous effort over the life cycle.

The clinical assessment of the adolescent and late adolescent personality has been considered from many perspectives. For example, in terms of ego functioning (Freud, 1923; Schlessinger and Robbins, 1983); identity formation (Erikson, 1958, 1968, 1969); personal autonomy (Richmond and Sklansky, 1984); object choice (Blos 1979); separation-individuation (Blos, 1967; Mahler, 1969; Isay, 1980); capacities for love and work (attributed to Freud by Erikson [1950, p. 229]); or play (Alexander, 1958); freedom to be uniquely creative (Jacques, 1980); and to be ordinarily productive or in a related way the capacity to observe and appreciate beauty in nature and the arts; varying degrees of resolution of the Oedipus complex; transformations of infantile narcissism (Kohut, 1966); cognitive capacities for abstract or formal thinking (Inhelder and Piaget, 1958; Dulit, 1972, 1983; Brockman, 1984) as well as the accretion of other new cognitive skills; expansion of social and linguistic skills; ethical and moral development in terms of an expanded superego (Hartmann and Loewenstein, 1962; Kernberg, 1987); and finally an increased capacity for tolerance of frustration, anxiety, and depression (Zetzel, 1965; Schlessinger and Robbins, 1983). In regard to this impressive array of assessment tools, it is remarkable that a definitive study of the personality of young adults has been relatively neglected in the psychoanalytic literature.

Among the many developmental transformations of late adolescence noted above and enumerated by Gould (1978, 1987) would be consolidation of the personality, diversion of energies to mastery of the drives, and successful manipulation of external reality. When these tasks have been successfully negotiated, it is possible to speak of a mature young adult personality. In contrast, pseudomaturity is a forced or premature development that has been stimulated by steady unrelenting pressures from a traumatic environment or the more catastrophic conditions of a death in the family, the tragedy of a divorce in the family, job loss, being passed over for advancement, or failure to gain admission to graduate or professional school. Even more dramatic in this regard are the precocious developments brought on by sobering war experiences. Most often, however, across various cultures there are the gradual and quietly imperceptible changes of growing up into adulthood under more ordinary conditions that family and friends hardly notice until some external event exposes those functionally operative adult qualities and characteristics.

Impulsiveness so common in adolescence gives way to more considered thinking and delayed action. Similarly, the impact of socialization processes becomes visible when called on by life experience, such as the responsible roles of citizen and procreator. Normal young parents, for example, relatively easily assume responsibility for their children, or in a more dramatic way, young nurses and doctors in hospital emergency rooms make life and death decisions in rapid succession.

Another example involves the political activists of the 1960s whose behavior then was characterized by militant street marches, sit-ins at university administration buildings, and antiwar demonstrations. These same individuals are seen now to have transformed their social responsibilities to professional areas while retaining a sharpened social consciousness (lawyers, doctors, homemakers, ministers, teachers, accountants, members of Congress, and entrepreneurial businesspeople). They were not so "co-opted" by the system as they had earlier feared, but the inexorable identification and socialization processes left significant developmental incremental changes in their wake.

The study of these growth processes which we are considering in developmental language, comes from the various disciplines of sociology, life-span developmental psychology research, psychoanalytic reconstruction in the analyses of

adults, direct observations of, and here in this work, psychoanalytic therapy with young adults. The language of the processes
associated with the acquisition of various roles (e.g., citizen,
procreator, creator, and provider) comes from the sociologists,
and from psychoanalysis comes the observation and concept
of internalization of qualities and characteristics that compose
the consolidated personality (Schafer, 1968). For all students
of human development it is important to learn from a wide
variety of disciplines, in order to approach a greater understanding of these very complex processes. The psychotherapeutic process also promotes the socialization of patients (Orne
and Wender, 1968).

Developmental processes and socialization processes impact
on young people simultaneously and are studied and described
by researchers from these two different disciplines. Development occurs over the entire course of life, and developmental
changes reflect biological, social, psychological, physical, and
historical issues. Biological issues also imply evolutionary assumptions. Mulitvariables interact and have a cumulative effect
(Featherman, 1983). While some of the same language is used,
the conceptualizations are very different and thus lead to divergent explanations and conclusions. As yet, there has not been
enough serious effort to integrate this growing body of knowledge. Solnit (1983) joins Bell (1968) and Peters (1985) in
pointing out the healthy effects of siblings on other siblings
and of siblings on parents to enhance their respective capacities to confront and resolve interpersonal, intrapsychic, and
various developmental hurdles and conflicts. Macooby (1984)
insists on a bidirectional process in which parents have to
change and adapt to the needs and personalities of their children. For example, one father reported that he was brought
up short when his seemingly innocent command to an 11-year-
old daughter was met by her response that she was "the boss
of herself." Mutual attachments, identifications, and empathic

resonances occur in the natural environment of a family. Companionship, rivalries, envy, jealousy, hatred, and reassurances contribute, Solnit (1983) says, to growth in constructive capacities for tolerance, regulation of tension, anticipation, planning, and adaptation.

Offer and Offer in their book *From Teenage to Young Manhood* (1975), describe three different pathways to adulthood: continuous growth, surgent growth, and tumultuous growth. These developmental routes were abstracted from survey tests and interviews with a homogenous group of young suburban men who were studied over a period of eight years. This study was more sociological than in-depth psychoanalytic psychology, even though brief interviews lend some clinical credibility and validity to the study. Their conclusion that inner turmoil is not a regular or necessary ingredient of the adolescent phase, in my opinion, is open to question when in-depth assessment almost invariably reveals the presence of inner conflicts (A. Freud, 1936; Blos, 1962). The experienced psychoanalytic clinician is forced to question the concept of continuous growth without conflict or symptoms. It seems a reasonable conclusion that some discontinuity and regression with symptom formation must be at the very least common in most individuals.

Emde (1985) also calls for integration of psychological data with sociological data in studying the progression from adolescence to adulthood. His emphasis is on the "transactional self," which develops out of the interaction with the social environment. He refers to the well-known example of marriage partners who successfully navigate the hazardous waters of adult intimacy by negotiation and other interactive patterns. These are daily issues that arise between marriage partners; for example, over their respective careers, how finances are managed, how leisure time is spent, or gratification of sexual desires. These are the multiform interactions with children of various ages who are involved in their own phase specific conflicts, which in turn induce destabilizing regressive reactivations of the parents' own childhood conflicts.

Sociological studies show that the middle class is fragmenting and is no longer so homogenous, and one of the reasons for this fragmentation process is attributed to the high rate of divorce in American families. In addition, families are dislocated from their families of origin, thereby losing important social support systems, and there are often no grandparents nearby to assist the young parents in processing their developmental tasks as young adults. Today there seem to be fewer young radicals or "anticonformists" who follow their own individualistic paths as described some years ago by Kenniston (1965, 1968) and the number of politically uncommitted seems to be larger—the reverse of the number of just a few decades ago. Even though another wave (though scattered and episodic) of student rebellion and public protest seems to be taking place again, the sociological scene of youth today is that they are more studious and too serious about their careers to enter into political activities that take away from their studies (Galatzer-Levy and Cohler, 1993). This is a sad commentary since it is to be deplored that so many young people who have the vote do not use it.

The internal psychological conditions that permit, facilitate, and ensure the dominance of the principles of continuity (Lichtenberg, 1984; Emde and Harmon, 1986) over discontinuity are part of what I want to emphasize in this chapter. What is meant by dominance of continuity is that development is considered to be a dynamic process of progressive and regressive movements, which in the optimal sense, proceed among a variety of possibilities toward adult or genital character formation. The genital character, as Reich (1949) originally described it, is the sum total of various developmental achievements. These include decathexis of the Oedipus complex and mastery of castration anxiety as manifested by the free capacity for orgastic discharge of sexual tension within which there has been integration of pregenital drives and the unfettered use of sublimation which allows for increased capacities for work and play. Reich's concept of the genital character was a good beginning in describing the composition of the young adult personality.

Freud (1905) in *Three Essays on the Theory of Sexuality* refers to normal sexual life as arising in a "convergence of the affectionate current and the sensual current, both being directed towards the sexual object and sexual aim" (p. 207). The last phase of sexual development according to Freud is when sexual aims are subordinated in the service of reproduction. However, it is not at all clear that the sole pathway to adult object love requires becoming a parent. In fact, there are many persons who remain single or childless and must be considered adult in every sense of the word. Yet another way of looking at the problem of deciding who is an adult is to conceptualize a variety of adult behaviors as derived from clinical observations. Abraham (1925) regarded a person's character as the "sum of his instinctual reactions towards his social environment" (p. 408), but that character is a changeable thing. Abraham (1925) made the point that the genital character is no longer ambivalent toward the genital organ of the heterosexual partner and is "relatively unnarcissistic" (p. 416). Even though Fenichel (1945) said that the genital character is an "ideal concept" (p. 496), it nevertheless has been a clinically useful concept to help describe what is included in a description of an adult character.

A thorough psychoanalytic assessment of young adults must take into account all those very important ego functions that Schlessinger and Robbins (1983) have emphasized: basic trust;

object constancy; dyadic object constancy; self-constancy; dyadic object relationship competence; dyadic reality processing; tolerance of and potential for mastery of frustration, anxiety, and depression; triadic object relationship competence; triadic reality processing; regression in the service of the ego; therapeutic split; self-analytic function; self-soothing function (Kohut, 1971); transformation of narcissism (Kohut, 1966); and finally the analyst's contributions to the analytic situation (Kohut, 1984). I shall not take up each and every one of these functions separately, since in any analysis virtually all of this list of ego functions should be addressed when they are in focus at one time or another. However, the capacity for a therapeutic split is an imperative since without it no psychoanalytic or psychotherapeutic process can take place.

SOCIALIZATION PROCESSES

Featherman (1983) considers socialization from a life-span perspective. Development occurs over the entire course of life and in general developmental changes reflect biological (including evolutionary assumptions), social, psychological, physical, and historical issues. Socialization, according to Featherman, refers "to the complex processes whereby an individual learns and modifies behavior, values, and emotions that are deemed appropriate by the community and larger society" (p. 10). These processes are also influenced by the demands placed on the learner at different periods of the life span. For example, the demands on children are different from those on adolescents and young adults. In adolescence and young adulthood, team sports can make a significant contribution to socialization processes since Butcher (1983) showed that adolescent girls' participation in intramural sports delivered improved physical and social competence and increased self-confidence. Sports permit the release of aggression and promote the development of lasting bonds of friendship, as well as the idealizing of peers and the demonizing of "enemies" (Solomon and Grunebaum, 1982).

The concept of the team as a family with bonds of empathic caring is heavily promoted in all sports, and especially in professional sports to create an atmosphere of horizontal affectional ties creating social competence, real unity, and cohesiveness that breeds success in a particular sport. Social competence is somewhat loosely defined, but Adams (1983) emphasizes capacities for empathy, a belief in the power of self-initiation (locus of control), and individual knowledge about appropriate emotional states for specific social contexts (social knowledge). There are certainly other activities similar to sports, such as participation in school orchestras, bands, choirs, theater, or language clubs, all of which involve the acquisition of skills that last a lifetime and at the same time produce a great deal of pleasure.

The psychological and developmental effects of the death of a parent in childhood were studied in the Parent Loss Project at the Institute for Psychoanalysis in Chicago (Fleming, 1963; Altschul, 1988). The patients who were analyzed by the group were found to be arrested in development and were typically unable to accomplish certain developmental tasks such as graduation from college, completion of a graduate degree, or maintenance of a successful relationship with a love object leading to marriage. The mourning work (Freud, 1917) had to be reinstated in the transference to unloosen the arrested development. From a sociological perspective, Fry (1983) has shown that cognitive, intellectual skills and social problem-solving competency are also seriously impaired when the father is absent, since the father normally provides a significant feedback in terms of cognitive–intellectual stimulation. The effects appear early and are cumulative in terms of social sensitivity and accuracy of labeling affects in others, understanding of social roles, and moral judgments. Moreover, father loss in childhood leads to specific deficits in late adolescence and young adulthood when decisions regarding career choices and object choices are being made (Brockman, 1988).

Stigmatization of the gay adolescent and young adult prevents normal socialization and instills a negative identity. In fact, the gay person may remain in the closet until a later age when it is permissible to attend gay social gatherings (Martin, 1982; Isay, 1986; Boxer, Cohler, Herdt, and Irwin, 1993) (see chapter 3).

Parsons and Platt (1972) refer to a "studentry" phase of development corresponding to late adolescence and young adulthood. Since the 1970s, advanced education in college and graduate schools has become increasingly necessary. Parsons and Platt (1972) list the socializing effects of the college experience: capacity to accept higher levels of achievement for self and others; requiring rational acceptance of authority and coordination of group efforts in agreed upon tasks; capacity to accept and participate in a more differentiated environment together with extensively pluralized courses of action. There is less slavish devotion to authority and more cognitive rationality, along with a dissolution and reordering of religious and societal values and standards. "The college student learns to locate a multiplicity of collective affiliations within a differentiated network, giving relevance to each affiliation and attributing to none an absolute commitment" (p. 253). Even more so today, student protests have focused on racism, intolerance toward gays, grading systems, depersonalization, and bureaucratization of the college culture and society at large, complicity of universities with the military–industrial complex, and a demand for greater expressiveness and participation in administrative policies.

Van Snippenburg and Vettehen (1992) described a group of "postadolescents" who have left the parental home but are not yet employed, nor have they established stable partnerships or a structured sense of social identity. They studied the cohort arriving at this age group in the 1970s, whom they found to be associated with liberal and postmaterialist causes, thus differing from those more conservative young adults who were settled in jobs, married, and had children. The contrasting 1980s cohort were influenced by the stagnation in the world economy but were less different in their political and social values from the more settled young adults. The rootlessness of the generations of the 1980s and 1990s was characterized by the fact they were not married or employed even though they were marriageable and employable. The old anchors of previous generations no longer held. Van Snippenburg and Vettehen postulate that these differences in the 1980s cohort were inversely related to the length of time they are exposed to the liberal and post-materialist values in the educational system. Conventional wisdom suggests that by a wide margin not all young married adults who are childless end up as liberal minded. But many young people in the 1990s seemed to be returning to the idealism of the 1960s in a political sense. Social stratifications, differentiation, and pluralization due to such things as age, specific occupations, multiple political groups, ethnic, gender, and sexual orientation are becoming more commonly studied aspects of modern social structure and social dynamics. For example, age stratification is an important element in the dynamics of society "influencing and being influenced by the behavior and attitudes of individual members of society" (Riley, Johnson, and Foner, 1972, p. xiv), as was seen in the 1960s when groups protesting against the Vietnam War influenced mainstream American culture and were influenced in turn. Luhmann's (1982) concept of a *centerless society* is that modern societies have changed from the more centered societies of the past, but are really not so fragile as one might expect from such compartmentalization, due to society's inherent resistance to disintegration. What keeps us together, Luhmann claims, is a "schematized contingency," "i.e., procedural rules for changing the status quo" (p. xix). These rules allow for changes to occur without serious fractures or dehumanization as described by Kenniston (1965, 1968). The multiple choices facing young adults in the 1990s, Luhmann claims, were not so destructive or destabilizing since there were many positive features to the multiple choices as there were negative ones.

Wertsch's comprehensive summary of Vygotsky's socialization processes (1985), details the uses of signs and signals as mediational means in both interpsychological and intrapsychological spheres. In this regard, the uses of language are grouped in terms of several opposites: the signaling function versus the significative function; social function versus individual function; communicative function versus intellectual function; indicative function versus symbolic function. Vygotsky's theory encompasses both animals and humans, since both communicate one to another, but humans alone use signs to "create new connections in the brain that constitute external influence" (Wertsch, 1985, p. 91). Signs, Vygotsky claimed, are always used as a "means of influencing others, and only later become a means of influencing oneself" (Wertsch, 1985, p. 92; Vygotsky, 1981, pp. 157–158). "The word's first function is its social function; and if we want to trace how it functions in the behavior of the individual, we must consider how it is used to function in social behavior" (Wertsch, 1985, p. 92; Vygotsky, 1981, pp. 157–158). Initially, words are used interpsychically to regulate the behavior of children. Vygotsky believed that language serves an emotional release function as well as being used for social contact. The communication is paired with the intellectual function, and it is clear from Vygotsky's point of view that content communication must go hand in hand with the stimulation of thinking and intellectual functions. The last pair of indicative and symbolization functions of speech refer to first orienting the listener to what is to follow and is "referential" (shades of Sorce and Emde's social referencing [1981]) and then the words can mediate meanings in abstract symbolic or metaphorical terms as in poetry, but also in ordinary speech where there is a degree of decontextualization involved. At about the age of 3, Vygotsky indicated, the development of egocentric speech begins, which is claimed to be an important forerunner of self-reflection and self-observation and hence the capacity for a therapeutic split. In adolescence, there is a further development of what Piaget calls "formal operations," or more generally, abstract thinking (Inhelder and Piaget, 1958), but Vygotsky's research pointed to the concomitant enhanced development of contextualized and decontextualized speech in the adolescent and on into adulthood.

THERAPEUTIC SPLIT

For the clinician, it is important to ascertain how well developed is a capacity for a therapeutic split (Sterba, 1934). By *therapeutic split* is meant the concept of a constructive dissociation within the patient's ego whereby the observing function is encouraged to separate off from the experiencing function. A therapeutic split is created by the joint efforts of the therapist and the patient within the therapeutic relationship. The therapist encourages the patient to observe what he is experiencing, and more particularly, to identify with the therapist's empathic observing capacities. The technique by which this construct and process is created, is through the liberal but judicious use of the plural pronouns. For example, the therapist might say: "Let us see what is going on in your relationship with your wife" (husband, boss, friends, parents, etc.), or "We can understand you better if we look more closely at what is going on here in our relationship." In other words, the patient is alerted to the possible presence of transferences that can be interpreted and understood. Young adults are more likely to have this capacity than the more junior adolescents, though (Brockman, 1984) some adolescents and even latency-aged children may already possess the capacity for a therapeutic split, thus making analytic work possible at an earlier age than was previously considered possible (Adatto, 1958; Chused, 1987a). Self-constancy, object constancy, self-observation, constructive self-criticism, together with the therapeutic split, provide the foundation for the young adult's self-analytic function (Schlessinger and Robbins, 1983). In other words, the personality of the young adult is more integrated and consolidated than is true of the average adolescent. The functional ego structures or capacities must be intact and reasonably resistant to massive regression, but be able to selectively regress in the service of the ego aims of the therapy. One of the important goals of therapy is the internalization of the self-analytic function. What is also important is that there be a certain degree of psychological mindedness and intellectual curiosity to construct a therapeutic split within the ego (Sterba, 1934), a process which the analyst and analysand construct together. In the initial phase, as Sterba recommended, liberal use of the plural pronouns *we*, *our*, and *us* fosters the development of a favorably convincing atmosphere of sympathetic interest. It is crucial in the early phase of analysis to sensitively launch the process through appropriate interpretations of initial anxieties and early transference reactions, ego regressions, and the emergence of disturbing unconscious contents through affectively laden fantasies, dreams, and free associations. It goes without saying that Freud's injunctions about abstinence (1915, 1919) are a prerequisite for the development of a viable therapeutic process and therapeutic relationship. Greenson (1967) referred to the working alliance, Zetzel and Meissner (1973) to the therapeutic alliance, and T. Benedek referred to the therapeutic relationship. All three terms describe the same phenomenon, a structured, split-off part of the personality that can effectively enter into a contract with the analyst for the common goal of relieving suffering, since it is psychic pain and a thirst for insight that really fuels the therapeutic process.

Mary was a young adult woman who was in the process of settling down in a marriage. She had two small children, but she was compelled by unconscious motives to be the big mamma to her brothers and sisters as well as her own widowed mother. Loaning them money and immersing herself in their various problems to help solve them was part of what she felt compelled to supply whenever anyone of them was in distress. She even took in her husband's employees when they were fired. She was hurt when neither siblings nor friends reciprocated her generosity. In the initial stages of her therapy she was very cautious and hesitant about making a commitment to therapy for fear she would have to reveal her unconscious rage at her father who had never been around when she was growing up. Interpretations were offered during the initial period to the effect that she was afraid of getting into her feelings about her father, especially since he had just died. She gradually relaxed enough in response to these initial interpretations to challenge my therapeutic style and raised pertinent questions about the contrasting therapeutic styles of her two previous therapists. In addition, she gained confidence in resisting her family's efforts to play on her guilt feelings about being more independent financially and emotionally. She continued to be generous but was more prudently realistic at the same time.

A young professional Jewish man was reluctant to use the couch since the passivity he experienced in the recumbent position evoked memories of a homosexual relationship he had engaged in during graduate school. That relationship had many meanings to him, as the later analysis uncovered, but the initial meaning was that he again longed for a compassionate, understanding relationship with a man that the homosexual relationship had supplied at a time when he very much needed it. What the analytic situation offered was an opportunity to work through his conflicts about his need for a tender, affectionate, and understanding relationship with a man. When this meaning was conveyed to him, his initial resistance was alleviated and he was better able to make use of the analytic process.

SEPARATION-INDIVIDUATION

The late adolescent phase of development (Brockman, 1984) is characterized by a reworking of those geographic but most importantly psychological efforts at separation from parents (Blos, 1967; Mahler, 1969; Mahler, Pine, and Bergman, 1975; Isay, 1980), specifically, separating from those residues of infantile ties and establishing a unique ego identity (Erikson, 1959; see chapter 2). One of the young adult's tasks in separating from the internalized relationship with the parents of his childhood involves establishing a new relationship with his parents and other authority figures in the sense of adult to adult, where give and take, mutual respect for differing points of view, abilities, talents, and interests abide. D. Levinson and his coworkers (1978) referred to the mentor role which a senior colleague has with a young adult some 8 to 15 years his junior and who is working to establish his own status as separate from that of his parents. It is more of a collegial atmosphere, where the senior person accepts and acknowledges his junior colleague's talents and competence and in doing so assists the young adult to separate from parents by providing a new object with whom he can identify and interact in a more adult way. He helps define the newly emerging professionalism of the junior person.

In the psychiatric and psychoanalytic specialties we are familiar with the situation of supervisors and supervisees. Here, the relationship is primarily a learning or preceptor situation. The novice must be able to regress in the service of the ego in the cognitive sphere in order to place himself in the position of the pupil so that he can be exposed to and familiarize himself with the intricate complexities of his chosen field (Kris, 1962). But without a stable degree of separateness, the learning alliance is not strong enough to permit the temporary and reversible regressive relationship with the supervisor-teacher. When there is a stable and healthy learning alliance, there is ample opportunity to learn the supervisor's technique but no less importantly to imitate and later identify with the supervisor through internalization of those values, ideals, and standards supervisor and supervisee together consider important. The supervisee internalizes the analyzing function of the supervisor which is combined with this same function from his training analyst, and out of this matrix constructs his own particular style of therapeutic technique.

Internalization and identity formation are taken up in the next chapter, but I want to emphasize that the mentor-supervisor facilitates the entire separation–individuation process. Moreover, analytic supervisees must learn about the psychological makeup of the opposite sex. It is often instructive if male supervisees learn about the psychological nature of their female patients from a female supervisor. Likewise, a similar rule applies to female supervisees learning about male patients from male supervisors. The reason for this arrangement is to facilitate the refinement of those uniquely sensitive and empathic skills in understanding gender related issues that are specific for men and women, since each individual is uniquely made up of a mixture of masculine and feminine qualities (see chapter 3). The transferences and countertransferences, as well as identifications and counteridentifications that arise in the learning situation, have been elaborated by Fleming and Benedek (1966) in their classic monograph, and need not be elaborated here. Levinson et al. (1978) correctly interpret the mentor relationship as a loving or libidinally charged one, with a predictable course of beginning and middle phases culminating in a natural ending phase, and a gradual diminution of the intensity that existed before. In the best of circumstances, ambivalences and competitive rivalries are avoided through analysis since in the psychoanalytic training program the candidate is required to be in analysis himself during a significant part of his supervisory work, and the supervisor must do his "homework" to provide the best possible environment for learning. As a case in point, the Freud–Jung relationship and collaboration suffered because of unanalyzed problems, notably unconscious homosexual conflicts and power struggles in their relationship.

The supervisor shares in the analytic candidate's ambitions, believes in him, and helps him to define his newly emerging identity. In a way, as Levinson et al. (1978) write, the supervisor-mentor is like a transitional figure who provides a constructive holding environment (Modell, 1976) within which the student's evolving analytic credentials, unique therapeutic style, and consolidation of those identificatory processes develop, leading to the construction of a professional self.

A case in point was Chekhov (Troyat, 1986; Yarmolinsky, 1973), the great Russian writer who on December 3, 1898, praised the young and unknown Gorky, who had idealized Chekhov in his letters. Chekhov wrote back with helpful suggestions about the writing craft, criticizing Gorky's facile overwriting. First he complimented him on his recognizable talent, but he then suggested that Gorky exercise restraint, because he found Gorky's prose monotonous. He admonished Gorky to be more parsimonious and less verbose in his descriptions.

> I'll begin by saying that in my opinion you lack restraint. You are like a spectator in a theater who expresses his enthusiasm so

unreservedly that he prevents himself and others from listening. This lack of restraint is particularly apparent in the descriptions of nature with which you interrupt dialogues; reading these descriptions, one wishes they were more compact, briefer—just two or three lines. Frequent mention of "bliss," "whispering," "velvety softness" and the like imparts a certain rhetorical and monotonous quality to these descriptions, and they chill, almost tire one. A lack of restraint is felt also in your depictions of women ("Malva," "on the Rafts"). And the love scenes. This is not breadth—a bold stoke of the brush—but simply a lack of restraint [Chekhov quoted in Yarmolinsky, 1973, pp. 320–321].

From the very first, there was an open advisory relationship corresponding to a mentor relationship between the two men. As is clear from the foregoing discussion, the young adult is involved in relating to other adults as mentors, but it must be remembered that relationships with other young adults as friends and peers assist the young adult also to learn much about separation issues, identifications, and intimacy.

RESOLUTION OF THE OEDIPUS COMPLEX

The third area of assessment is the task of determining the degree of relative resolution, "re-solution" or new solution of the oedipal conflict. In a clinical instance of a 25-year-old man, a pathological lag had occurred in the relinquishment of infantile sexual claims on the oedipal object so that the entire personality suffered. What was somewhat spared, as is so often the case, was a precocious and uneven development of specialized and outstanding intellectual achievements. Abstract thinking, mathematical and logical problem solving, and an avid interest in ancient literature presented far less conflictual opportunities for regression and thus were spared significant loss of function. But extensive investments in pregenital fixations were foci for

very painful transference reenactments of early object deprivations and traumatic overstimulations. There were repeated
bouts of bulimia and ineffective impulse control requiring repeated reassurances about fears of abandonment, overwhelming loneliness, and feelings of worthlessness. These regressive
episodes were precipitated by separations from the therapy,
including scheduled vacations, weekends, and breaks in the
empathic bond of the therapeutic relationship. There was serious erosion of self and object constancy and separation–individuation developmental achievements. In this clinical
instance, there was a failure of the processes of continuity and
consolidation. Energies for engagement in loving relationships, competitive play, and for use with creative talents, were
seriously hampered.

What is emphasized in this brief vignette is one way of describing the disruption of growth in the personality of a young
adult. This young man was highly motivated to achieve his
dream of certain career goals, and a thorough working through
of his unconscious conflicts led to greater comfort in intimacy
and freed up energies to be used in creative work and putting
his intellectual talents to good use.

In another young man, intense murderous conflicts with his
father were reenacted in the transference as coldness and withdrawal, which were mainly due to failures in empathic connectedness to the analyst, some of which were rarely due to
countertransference issues. The nature of his conflict early on
was predominately dyadic, and interfered with an already be-
sieged object constancy, and most importantly from the clinical
standpoint the development of a fuller, phallic investment in
his work and marriage. He began to realize some of his professional potentials after he began to address the traumatic aban-
donments by his parents and work through some of the
transference meanings of those early childhood experiences.

He then entered into an analytic relationship that could be characterized as triadic and competitive.

A young adult woman's first three diagnostic sessions were filled with a continuous, angry diatribe directed at her father. Her anger was unrelenting and unforgiving for his bullying, self-centeredness regarding both her and her mother. As an example of his brutish, overbearing penuriousness, she described the story of how her father refused to call a cab and made her mother walk several blocks to the hospital when she was in labor. In terms of developing adolescent sexuality and intellectual capacities, she felt unresponded to and unconfirmed. She was minimally encouraged by him to become a nurse. In late adolescence she felt strong enough to break away from this unrealistic identity and career choice to finish at the top of her law school class and enter a prestigious international law firm. However, her object choice was distorted and pathologically influenced due to unresolved oedipal issues. She was only dimly aware of her rivalry with her mother, which she kept repressed through her disgust and anger at her father's bellicose failures to respond appropriately to her during her oedipal phase.

In a third vignette, a 24-year-old professional woman was obsessed with men, even though she had just gotten married. She was afraid she would turn out like her mother, who had divorced when the patient was 6 months old, and her grandmother, whose husband had abandoned her. Her subsequent relationship with her father was limited, but she had very lively fantasies about him, especially after she had visited him in his apartment as a latency and preadolescent girl. A major part of the early phase of her analysis was consumed with working through the neurotic configurations of those behaviors and attitudes in her personality which stood in the way of the development of a triadic transference. For example, she externalized and displaced the transference onto men at work; she concentrated on feminist issues as if her analyst were sexist, and she identified with her mother's and grandmother's position as wronged and abandoned women. In fact, as it was later learned, the great grandmother was also abandoned by her husband, making a not so rare three-generation sequence. Adolescent defenses consisting of sham fights with her analyst early on served the purpose of keeping the erotic father transference from emerging. She used vacations and other interruptions as a way of cooling and delaying the deepening of the analytic process.

Another young adult woman lost her mother at age 14 just at a time when she needed her mother to help her negotiate the developmental tasks of adolescence. Instead, she was thrown together with her father, who did his best to raise her, but his emphasis was on intellectual, artistic, and cultural pursuits. Her complaints on entering analysis consisted of depression, an inability to finish her dissertation, and a marked failure to effect a lasting relationship with a suitable man. In fact, she acted out sexually with a variety of married men. Separation issues and unfinished mourning characterized the first period of the analysis, especially in terms of a massive resistance against the development of a utilizable transference. Intellectual defenses and nonstop associations kept her analyst at bay, as well as her unconscious conflicts accompanying her early adolescent "oedipal" victory. A notable change took place in her analysis when she began to experience the significance of her transference relationship with her analyst. This occurred in connection with a summer vacation interruption. She was tearful and spontaneously associated to the mother's death. At the same time she began to seriously question her sexual behavior and for the first time independently assumed more restraint in that area of her life.

A young adult man's manifest negative Oedipus complex did not appear in the transference until the patient's mother died rather suddenly and unexpectedly about nine months into the analysis. His wish to please me and his father and replace the mother (and a female patient of mine that he knew), was acted out in his efforts to care for his father in the same fashion as the mother had done while she was alive. His fantasies and dreams confirmed this formulation. He had to remain single in order to be available for his father's needs. As this transference was interpreted and worked through he was able to extricate himself from this self-sacrificing life. Early in life, the father was "absent" psychologically speaking and the patient was overinvolved with his mother throughout childhood, a situation similar to what Bibring has described (1953). A fuller examination of this case is taken up in chapter 4.

When there has been a working through of the major elements of the Oedipus complex, as implicitly demanded in the foregoing clinical vignettes, through systematic and successful psychoanalytic interpretation of the transference neurosis, the personality of the young adult can become more structurally well defined (Richmond and Sklansky, 1984). In Freud's paper "The Dissolution of the Oedipus Complex" (1924), the assertion is made that the Oedipus complex is demolished by the threat of castration. But, as Freud himself pointed out, if repression is the only mechanism involved, then the Oedipus complex "persists in an unconscious state in the id and will later manifest its pathogenic effect" (p. 177) on the personality, as implied in the case vignettes described above. Many neurotic young adult patients with structured personalities reveal the presence of unresolved oedipal conflicts when subjected to psychoanalytic inquiry. Normal development, though, implies that a major reorganization has taken place in the personality of young adults when there has been a naturally occurring and gradual decathexis of libidinized internal object relationships.

What is critical in this developmental task is the relinquishment of infantile and adolescent sexual claims on oedipal objects. This is what is meant by the concept of a resolution or re-working of the Oedipus complex. Psychoanalysis facilitates this process in patients when these conflicts are reenacted in the transference neurosis and interpreted in a timely fashion (Schlessinger and Robbins, 1983). Resolution of the Oedipus complex in women follows a different path. The task for women is made more difficult since a primary attachment to their mothers persists into adulthood and is characterized by much mutual ambivalence and conflict (Deutsch, 1944; Chodorow, 1978, 1989a,b). Psychoanalysis of young adult women and reconstruction of the young adult period from the analysis of adults confirms this view and that of Blos (1962) to the effect that separation from her mother is the "major task" of the adolescent girl.

CAREER CHOICE

A young man of 21 struggled to attain enough inner stability to settle on a career. He dreamed of becoming an entrepreneur and running his own business. At first he was a home builder's assistant, but tiring of the long hours and little pay, he started to drive a cab while attending night school to finish his college degree. For a while he worked for his father as a manufacturer's representative. Nothing seem to click for him and he continued to struggle. It was only after significant analytic work dealing with his repressed conflicts with his cold and indifferent father was he able to extricate himself from the web of a regressive and submissive relationship with his father and with me in the transference. What made all this possible involved experiencing me in the transference as the father who had repeatedly set him up for frustration. A murderous rage emerged, was interpreted, and worked through. As the analytic process allowed for a reexperiencing of the nuclear conflict within the transference, he began at first to identify with me in rather subtle ways in terms of clothing and a common avocational interest. This led to an open but friendly competition. He wanted to do me one better. The analysis then took on a different caste of collaborating with me in trying to construct the origins of his neurotic paralysis in finding suitable work, and a mutually satisfying heterosexual relationship with an appropriate young woman. He found a niche for himself in one of the financial markets and became reasonably successful in that rather competitive field.

SUMMARY

In summary, an informed clinical psychoanalytic assessment of the young adult must address the relative degree of consolidation of the personality. What is involved in consolidation are eight different manifest and latent variables in the transition from adolescence to young adulthood. They are: choosing an adult sexual object; consolidation of sexual and gender identities; expansion of certain ego functions that are relatively free of conflict, or in self psychological terms, the self is more cohesive; freeing up of energies for creative and productive work; intimate relations with peers, older and younger persons become less self-serving and self-aggrandizing; a harmonious character structure; enhanced ethical and moral values and standards; and being prepared for parenthood. Instinctual drives are more successfully mastered to allow for a greater command of external reality. From a sociological perspective, the transition to young adulthood is facilitated by interaction with others in a bidirectional process. Within a family structure, attachments, identifications, and empathic resonances help to master rivalries, jealousies, envies, and hatreds. The result is improved regulation of tensions and greater adaptation to each other. Discontinuities and derailments of this optimal process do occur with traumatic and disastrous results. Some clinical vignettes are given to illustrate these biopsychosociological processes.

REFERENCES

Abraham, K. (1925), Character formation on the genital level of the libido. In: *Selected Papers of Karl Abraham, M.D.*, tr. D. Bryan & A. Strachey. London: Hogarth Press, 1948.

Adams, G. R. (1983), Social competence during adolescence: Social sensitivity, locus of control, empathy, and peer popularity. *J. Youth & Adol.*, 12:203–211.

Adatto, C. (1958), Ego reintegration observed in analysis of late adolescents. *Internat. J. Psycho-Anal.*, 39:172–177.

——— (1980), Late adolescence to early adulthood. In: *The Course of Life*, Vol. 2, S. I. Greenspan & G. H. Pollock. ed. Washington, DC: National Institute of Mental Health.

Alexander, F. (1958), A contribution to the theory of play. *Psychoanal. Quart.*, 27:175–193.

Altschul, S. (1988), *Childhood Bereavement and Its Aftermath*. Madison, CT: International Universities Press.

Arnstein, R. L. (1989), Overview of normal transition to young adulthood. *Adolescent Psychiatry*, 16:127–141. Chicago: University of Chicago Press.

Bell, R. Q. (1968), A reinterpretation of the direction of effects in studies of socialization. *Psycholog. Rev.*, 75:81–93.

Benedek, T. (1959), Parenthood as a developmental phase. *J. Amer. Psychoanal. Assn.*, 7:389–417.

——— (1970), Parenthood during the life cycle. In: *Parenthood: Its Psychology and Psychopathology*, ed. E. J. Anthony & T. Benedek. Boston: Little. Brown, pp. 185–206.

Bibring, G. (1953), On the passing of the Oedipus complex in a matriarchal family setting. In: *Drives, Affects and Behavior: Essays in Honor of Marie Bonaparte*, ed. R. M. Loewenstein. New York: International Universities Press, pp. 278–284.

Block, J., with Haan, M. (1971), *Lives Through Time*. Berkeley, CA: Bancroft.

Blos, P. (1962), *On Adolescence: A Psychoanalytic Interpretation*. New York: Free Press.

——— (1967), The second individuation process of adolescence. *The Psychoanalytic Study of the Child*, 22:162–186. New York: International Universities Press.

—— (1979), *Adolescent Passage.* New York: International Universities Press.

Boxer, A. M., Cohler, B. J., Herdt, G., & Irwin, F. (1993), The study of gay and lesbian teenagers: Life course, "coming out" and well-being. In: *Handbook of Clinical Research and Practice with Adolescents,* ed. P. H. Tolan & B. J. Cohler. New York: John Wiley, pp. 249–280.

Brockman, D. D. (1984), *Late Adolescence: Psychoanalytic Studies.* New York: International Universities Press.

—— (1988), Preadolescence and early adolescence. In: *Child Bereavement and Its Aftermath,* ed. S. Altschul. Madison, CT: International Universities Press, pp. 351–376.

Butcher, J. (1983), Socialization of adolescent girls into physical activity. *Adolescence,* 18:753–766.

Chodorow, N. (1978), *The Reproduction of Mothering.* Berkeley: University of California Press.

—— (1989a), What is the relation between the psychoanalytic psychology of women and psychoanalytic feminism? *The Annual of Psychoanalysis,* 17: 215–242. Hillsdale, NJ: Analytic Press.

—— (1989b), *Feminism and Psychoanalytic Theory.* New Haven, CT: Yale University Press.

Chused, J. F. (1987a), Psychoanalysis of the young adult: Theory and technique. *J. Amer. Psychoanal. Assn.,* 35:175–187.

—— (1987b), Idealization of the analyst by the young adult. *J. Amer. Psychoanal. Assn.,* 35:839–859.

—— (1988), Transference neurosis in child analysis. *The Psychoanalytic Study of the Child,* 43:51–81. New Haven, CT: Yale University Press.

Connell, J. P., & Furman, W. (1984), The study of transitions. In: *Continuities and Discontinuities in Development,* ed. R. Emde & R. J. Harmon. New York: Plenum, pp. 153–173.

Deutsch, H. (1944), *The Psychology of Women: A Psychoanalytic Interpretation,* Vols. 1 & 2. New York: Grune & Stratton.

Dulit, E. (1972), Adolescent thinking à la Piaget: The formal stage. *J. Youth & Adol.,* 1: 281–301.

—— (1983), Cognitive development in adolescence: Clinical update. *Adolescent Psychiatry,* 1:2–7. Chicago: University of Chicago Press.

Eisenstadt, S. N. (1956), *From Generation to Generation.* Glencoe, IL: Free Press, 1971.

Emde, R. N. (1985), From adolescence to mid life: Remodeling the structure of adult development. *J. Amer. Psychoanal. Assn.,* 33:59–112.

—— Harmon, R. J., Eds. (1984), *Continuities and Discontinuities in Development.* New York: Plenum.

Erikson, E. H. (1950), *Childhood and Society.* New York: W. W. Norton.

—— (1958), *Young Man Luther.* New York: W. W. Norton.

—— (1959), Identity and the Life Cycle. *Psychological Issues,* Monogr. 1. New York: International Universities Press.

—— (1968), *Identity: Youth and Crisis*. New York: W. W. Norton.

—— (1969), *Ghandi's Truth*. New York: W. W. Norton.

Featherman, D. L. (1983), Life-span perspectives in social science research. In: *Life-Span Development and Behavior*, ed. P. B. Baltes & O. G. Brim, Jr. New York: Academic Press, pp. 1–57.

Fenichel, O. (1945), *The Psychoanalytic Theory of Neurosis*. New York: W. W. Norton.

Fleming, J. (1963), The evolution of a research project in psychoanalysis. In: *Counterpoint: Libidinal Object and Subject*, ed. H. S. Gaskill. New York: International Universities Press, pp. 75–105.

—— Benedek, T. (1966), *Psychoanalytic Supervision*. New York: International Universities Press.

Fountain, G. (1961), Adolescent into adult: An inquiry. *J. Amer. Psychoanal. Assn.*, 9:417–433.

Freud, A. (1936), *The Ego and the Mechanisms of Defense*. New York: International Universities Press, 1966.

Freud, S. (1905), Three Essays on the Theory of Sexuality. *Standard Edition*, 7:123–243. London: Hogarth Press, 1953.

—— (1915), Observations on transference love. *Standard Edition*, 12:159–171. London: Hogarth Press, 1958.

—— (1917), Mourning and melancholia. *Standard Edition*, 14:237–258. London: Hogarth Press, 1957.

—— (1919), Lines of advance in psycho-analytic therapy. *Standard Edition*, 17:157–165. London: Hogarth Press, 1955.

—— (1923), The Ego and the Id. *Standard Edition*, 19:1–59. London: Hogarth Press, 1961.

—— (1924), The dissolution of the Oedipus complex. *Standard Edition*, 19:171–179. London: Hogarth Press, 1961.

Fry, P. S. (1983), Father absence and defects in children's social, cognitive development: Implications for intervention and training. *J. Psychiat. Eval.*, 5:113–120.

Galatzer-Levy, R. M., & Cohler, B. (1993), *The Essential Other*. New York: Basic Books.

Gould, R. L. (1978), *Transformations: Growth and Change in Adult Life*. New York: Simon & Schuster.

—— (1987), Clarification of the normative tasks in the transition between adolescence and young adulthood: Ages 17 to 23. Presentation at the meeting of the American Society for Adolescent Psychiatry in Chicago, May 1987.

Greenson, R. (1967), *The Technique and Practice of Psychoanalysis*, Vol. 1. New York: International Universities Press.

Hartmann, H. (1950), Comments on the psychoanalytic theory of the ego. *The Psychoanalytic Study of the Child*, 5:74–96. New York: International Universities Press.

—— (1952), The mutual influences of the ego and the id. *The Psychoanalytic Study of the Child*, 7:9–30. New York: International Universities Press.

—— (1955), Notes on the theory of sublimation. *The Psychoanalytic Study of the Child*, 10:109–129. New York: International Universities Press.

—— (1958), *Ego Psychology and the Problem of Adaptation*, tr. D. Rapaport. New York: International Universities Press.

—— Loewenstein, R. M. (1962), Notes on the superego. *The Psychoanalytic Study of the Child*, 17:42–81. New York: International Universities Press.

Holland, N. (1985), *The I*. New Haven, CT: Yale University Press.

Inhelder, B., & Piaget, P. (1958), *The Growth of Logical Thinking*. New York: Basic Books.

Isay, R. A. (1980), Late adolescence: The second separation stage of adolescence. In: *The Course of Life*, Vol 2, ed. S. I. Greenspan & G. H. Pollock. Washington DC: National Institute of Mental Health, pp. 453–467.

—— (1986), The development of sexual identity in homosexual men. *The Psychoanalytic Study of the Child*, 41:467–489. New Haven, CT: Yale University Press.

Jacobson, E. (1964), *The Self and the Object World*. New York: International Universities Press.

Jacques, E. (1980), The mid-life crisis. In: *The Course of Life*, Vol. 3, ed. S. I. Greenspan & G. H. Pollock. Washington, DC: National Institute of Mental Health, pp. 1–23.

Josselson, R. (1989), Identity formation in adolescence: Implications for young adulthood. *Adol. Psychiatry*, 16:142–154. Chicago: University of Chicago Press.

Kenniston, K. (1965), *The Uncommitted*. New York: Dell/Delta.

—— (1968), *Young Radicals*. New York: Harcourt, Brace, & Jovanovich.

Kernberg, O. (1975), *Borderline Conditions and Pathological Narcissism*. New York: Jason Aronson.

—— (1987), Restructuring the superego and ego ideal. *J. Amer. Psychoanal. Assn.*, 36:1005–1029.

Kohut, H. (1966), Forms and transformations of narcissism. *J. Amer. Psychoanal. Assn.*, 14:243–272.

—— (1971), *The Analysis of the Self*. New York: International Universities Press.

—— (1984), *How Does Analysis Cure?* ed. A. Goldberg with P. Stepansky. Chicago: University of Chicago Press.

Kris, E. (1962), *Psychoanalytic Explorations in Art*. New York: International Universities Press.

Levinson, D. J., Arrow, C. N., Klein, E. B., Levinson, M. H., & McGee, B. (1978), *The Seasons of a Man's Life*. New York: Ballantine.

Lichtenberg, J. (1984), Continuities and transformations between infancy and adolescence. In: *Late Adolescence: Psychoanalytic Studies*, ed. D. D. Brockman. New York: International Universities Press.

Luhmann, N. (1982), *The Differentiation of Society,* tr. S. Holmes & C. Larmore. New York: Columbia University Press.

Macooby, E. E. (1984), Socialization and developmental change. *Child Develop.,* 55:317–328.

Mahler, M. (1969), *Human Symbiosis and the Vicissitudes of Individuation,* Vol. 1. New York: International Universities Press.

————— Pine, F., & Bergman, A. (1975), *The Psychological Birth of the Human Infant.* New York: Basic Books.

Marcia, J. E. (1980), Identity in adolescence. In: *Handbook of Adolescent Psychology,* ed. J. Adelson. New York: John Wiley, pp. 159–187.

Martin, A. D. (1982), Learning to hide: The socialization of the gay adolescent. *Adol. Psychiatry,* 10:52–65. Chicago: University of Chicago Press.

Modell, A. (1976), The "holding environment" and the therapeutic action of psychoanalysis. *J. Amer. Psychoanal. Assn.,* 24:285–307.

Offer, D., & Offer, J. B. (1975), *From Teenage to Young Manhood.* New York: Basic Books.

Orne, M. T., & Wender, P. H. (1968), Anticipatory socialization for psychotherapy: Method and rationale. *Amer. J. Psychiatry,* 124:1202–1212.

Parsons, T., & Platt, G. M. (1972), *Higher Education and Changing Socialization in Ageing and Society,* Vol. 3, ed. M. W. Riley, M. Johnson, & A. Foner. New York: Russell Sage Foundation, pp. 236–291.

Peters, J. F. (1985), Adolescents as socialization agents to parents. *Adolescence,* 20:921–933.

Rapaport, D., & Gill, M. (1959), Five metapsychological points of view. *Internat. J. Psycho-Anal.,* 40:153–162.

Reich, W. (1949), *Character Analysis.* New York: Orgone Institute Press.

Richmond, M. B., & Sklansky, M. A. (1984), Structural change in adolescence. In: *Late Adolescence: Psychoanalytic Studies,* ed. D. D. Brockman. New York: International Universities Press, pp. 97–121.

Riley, M. W., Johnson, M., & Foner, A. (1972), *Ageing and Society.* New York: Russell Sage Foundation.

Schafer, R. (1968), *Aspects of Internalization.* New York: International Universities Press.

Schlessinger, N., & Robbins, F. P. (1983), *A Developmental View of the Psychoanalytic Process.* New York: International Universities Press.

Solnit, A. (1983), The sibling experience. *The Psychoanalytic Study of the Child,* 38:281–284. New Haven, CT: Yale University Press.

Solomon, L., & Grunebaum, H. (1982), Stages in social development: Friendship and peer relations. *Hillside J. Clin. Psychiatry,* 4:95–126.

Sorce, J. F., & Emde, R. N. (1981), Mother's presence is not enough. *Develop. Psychol.,* 17:737–745.

Spiegel, L. (1961), Disorder and consolidation in adolescence. *J. Amer. Psychoanal. Assn.,* 9:406–416.

Sterba, R. (1934), The fate of the ego in analytic therapy. *Internat. J. Psycho-Anal.*, 15:117–126.
Troyat, H. (1986), *Chekhov,* tr. M. H. Heim. New York: Dutton.
Vaillant, G. E. (1977), *Adaptation to Life.* Boston: Little, Brown.
Van Snippenburg, L. B., & Vettehen, P. G. J. H. (1992), Dutch youth in transition to adulthood: Differential changes in their political and sociocultural values since the 1970's. *J. Youth & Adol.*, 21:573–591.
Vygotsky, L. S. (1960), *The Development of Higher Mental Functions.* Moscow: Izdatel'stvo Akademii Pedagogicheskikh.
———— (1981), The genesis of higher mental functions. In: *The Concept of Activity in Soviet Psychology,* ed. J. V. Wertsch. Armonk, NY: M. E. Sharpe, pp. 144–188.
Wertsch, J. V. (1985), *Vygotsky and the Social Formation of Mind.* Cambridge, MA: Harvard University Press.
Wolf, E., Gedo, J., & Terman, D. (1972), On the adolescent process as a transformation of the self. *J. Youth & Adol.*, 1:257–272.
Wolf, E. S. (1982), Adolescence: Psychology of the self and selfobjects. *Adol. Psychiatry,* 10:171–181. Chicago: University of Chicago Press.
Yarmolinsky, A. (1973), *Letters of Anton Chekhov,* tr. L. Solotaroff. New York: Viking Press, pp. 320–321.
Zetzel, E. (1965), Depression and the incapacity to bear it. In: *Drives, Affects, Behav.,* 2:342–274.
———— Meissner, W. W. (1973), *Basic Concepts in Psychoanalytic Psychiatry.* New York: Basic Books.

Chapter 2

Identity

A REVIEW OF THE LITERATURE

Etymologically, the word *identity* is derived from the Latin *idem* and the suffix *tas* or *tratem*. The noun expresses "the quality or condition of being the same in substance, composition, nature, properties, or in particular qualities under consideration; absolute or essential sameness; oneness" (*Compact Oxford English Dictionary*).

The concept of identity in psychoanalysis has been neglected in recent years (Gray, 1990), and remains unintegrated into the main body of psychoanalytic theory and clinical practice. Erikson (1956) popularized *identity* as a psychosocial and developmental term—*identity crises* and *identity diffusion*–to describe occurrences in late adolescents and young adults. These problems commonly occur late in the college career, after graduation, or for those who entered business without attending college or technical school when career choice and sexual object choice are experienced as overwhelming developmental tasks. Parent loss and other traumatic overstimulating, abusive experiences in childhood, whether sexual or physical, are risk factors leading to vertical splitting in the ego that in turn gives rise to clinically observable splits in identity (Shengold, 1980). The phase specific task of this transitional period of development, according to Erikson's life cycle schemata (1959), is intimacy versus isolation; for example, when some young people

35

are so frightened by the prospect of initiating intimacy that they withdraw from normal socializing with others, while others' efforts to socialize result in repeated failure and lead to increasing disappointment and disillusionment. For Erikson (1982) identity formation is:

> [A]n evolving configuration—a configuration that gradually integrates constitutional givens, idiosyncratic libidinal needs, favored capacities, significant identifications, effective defenses, successful sublimations, and consistent roles . . . [identity emerges only from a] mutual adaptation of individual potentials, technological world views, and religious and political ideologies [1982, p. 76].

Erikson's approach is loosely sociopsychological, and contains some very seminal ideas that are clinically useful.

In the psychoanalytic literature, the term *identity* was first used by Tausk (1919) in referring to the newborn's primary or innate narcissism associated with finding pleasure in its own body. This is a process which is repeated while shared pleasure and sameness with caretakers are discovered and established, as well as a process of psychological separateness in the form of precursors of the process of differentiation of the self from caretakers. Erikson (1956) proposed the concept of *identity* as a psychosocial or epigenetic term, which he described as evolving from all the constitutional givens, combined with libidinal needs, specific gifts, significant identifications, specific defenses, sublimations, and consistent roles in the synthesis and resynthesis of the ego. Erikson's purpose was to include the ego's conscious, preconscious, unconscious, and synthesizing activities in identity formation as well as a solid connection with group ideals. He permitted a certain conceptual looseness, but his concept grew out of his broad cultural interests, his observations of both healthy and psychologically ill young people, as well as social anthropological observations and comparative education. Erikson (1956) asserted that identity "connotes both a persistent sameness within oneself (self-sameness) and a persistent sharing of some kind of essential character with others" (p. 57). Like Tausk, Erikson (1959) said that identity's "roots go back all the way to the first self-recognition: in the baby's earliest exchange of smiles there is something of a self-realization coupled with a mutual recognition" (pp. 113–114).

Kramer (1955; Panel, 1958) conceptualized identity as related to separateness and an "awareness of being an entity separate and distinct from all others" (Panel, 1958, p. 133)—what one is and what one is not. A person engages in a series of decisions to be something and not be something else. In the same panel discussion, Greenacre (Panel, 1958) went a step further by saying that identity formation is brought about by a process of observing, comparing, and contrasting oneself with another person. The face and genitals are the prime areas of the body used in making these observations, which take place mainly in the phallic–oedipal period, though there is some "preliminary working form during the anal phase" (p. 625). She also said identity may change over the course of life in conjunction with maturational and bodily changes. Jacobson (Panel, 1958) emphasized the sameness as well as the differences between self and nonself. In addition, she felt that self representation was not the same as identity, which "depends on the effectiveness of the synthesizing, organizing functions of the ego. . . . The objective process of normal identity formation finds reflection at any stage of development in the normal subjective feeling of identity" (Jacobson, 1964, p. 27). Jacobson concluded that identity formation encompasses "man's complicated instinctual development, the slow maturation of his ego, his uneven superego formation, and the intricate vicissitudes of those object relations and identifications with his family and social milieu upon which his individual personal, cultural, social adult life in and with his environment is founded" (1964, p. 32). Bernstein (1963) differentiated between sense of identity and identity. For him sense of identity is a "conviction of the reality of one's own existence based on the ego's capacity to experience excitation" whereas identity is a "synthesis of the ego's perceptions of the self." L. Grinberg and R. Grinberg (1966) conceptualized identity as originating from a process of "continuous interaction between three links of integration: the spatial link, the temporal link, and the social link" (p. 53). By spatial link, they meant the relation between different aspects of the self including the body self "maintaining its cohesion and enabling comparison and contrast with objects; it tends to the self/nonself differentiation, i.e. individuation" (p. 55). By temporal link is meant the acquisition of various representations of the self over time which produces self-sameness. The social link refers to the process of identification with certain qualities and characteristics of objects. Patients come to analysis to consolidate their respective identities. The analytic setting provides the opportunity for projections and regressions in the transference so that certain pathological experiences can be relived, understood, reconstructed, and worked through. Thus, tiny elements of identity can coalesce to form a new more stable sense of self or identity. L. and R. Grinberg (1974) also considered identity in terms of the psychoanalytic process.

Wheelis (1958, 1959) conceived of identity "as a coherent sense of self" (p. 19), and particularly in terms of an ego ideal function. He defined identity as possessing goals which in turn are defined by values. In fact, he said that identity is founded on "those values which are at the top of the hierarchy—the beliefs, faiths and ideals which integrate and determine subordinate values" (1958, p. 200). Institutional values, he says, are particularly vulnerable to the massive and rapid changes wrought by the mechanics of an instrumental process in industrialized societies which inexorably erodes institutional value systems in Western cultures. Wheelis said: "Identity is not, therefore, to be found; it is to be created and achieved" (1958, p. 205), presumably through newly adopted values and goals which are reorganized into new identities.

Kernberg (1980) believed that the concept of self appears as an integration of a number of self representations during the oedipal and latency periods and at the same time good and bad self representations are integrated into an ego identity. As object constancy is established ego identity "is further consolidated" (p. 99). Conflicts concerning identity have to do with failures of the integration of good and bad representations as well as idealized and sadistic precursors of the superego. Kernberg (1987a,b) investigated the role of the superego in identity formation and its deterioration under group pressures as they are applied to young adult psychoanalytic candidates and graduates alike. Holland's (1985) study of identity theory is an attempt to encompass all of psychoanalysis into a general theory of the mind, and in addition he includes the neurophysiological concept of feedback mechanisms. He proposes a sixth metapsychological point of view to complement Rapaport and Gill's (1959) classic paper which attempts to organize psychoanalytic theoretical assumptions along five points of view (topographic, structural, economic, dynamic, and genetic). Holland suggests an additional personal or identity principle. He conceives of the "I" as agent, as a consequence, and as a representation.

> Very briefly, I act forth into the world from myself as agent (A) of what the world acts back onto me, so that I am a consequence (C) of what the world does both on its own and in response to my agency. My I initiates feedback but is also the consequence of the feedback it initiates. One can spell out those feedbacks as: expectation (E), what I am habituated to seek in the time-stream of my experience; defense (D), what I will admit into myself from the world; fantasy (F), what I project out into the

world; transformation (T), the meanings outside of time that I make my experience into [p. xi].

The "I" is also a representation (R) as well. According to Holland, the "I" is a theme and variations; both a constant and something that changes over time. Sexual and gender identity are not internally determined alone, since there are powerful stimuli in the infant's and child's environment that strongly influence the outcome of gender identity.

Marcia (1980) construes identity "as a self structure—an internal, self-constructed, dynamic organization of drives, abilities, beliefs, and an individual history" (p. 159). It "refers to an existential position, to an inner organization of needs, abilities, and self-perceptions as well as to a sociopolitical stance" (p. 159). Marcia conceptualizes identity as a self structure and gives support to Erikson's view of identity as composed of substructures located within the ego. However, these dynamic modes of functioning seem more like character types than either self structures or substructures of the ego. There are four general types: identity achievement; foreclosure; identity diffusion; and moratorium, that are defined by the presence or absence of a crisis and commitment to a vocation and an ideology. These groupings of personality styles provide the researcher with a rich array of possibilities with which to study identity in terms of anxiety level, self-esteem, authoritarianism, moral reasoning, autonomy, styles of cognition, and college behavior patterns. Marcia's studies have been confirmed by Adams, Ryan, Hoffman, Dobson, and Nielsen (1984).

The term *identity achievements* applies to those individuals who have worked their way through a decision-making process and are actively pursuing vocational and ideological goals. People to whom the term *foreclosures* applies differ from the previous category in that their career and ideological goals have been chosen for them. Neither group shows evidence of a crisis.

People to whom the term *identity diffusions* applies have not settled on either vocational or ideological goals. People who are actively struggling with career and ideological goals and values and are in the midst of an identity crisis, come in the category *moratoriums*. There are pathological and healthy variants among these identity groupings, save for those in the identity achievements group who seem to correspond to the normal or continuous growth group (Offer and Offer, 1975) and are characterized as "strong, self-directed, and highly adaptive" (p. 161). Students in the diffusion category are most affected by "peer pressure conformity, whereas identity-achievement students were most likely to report engaging in conformity behavior for achievement gains" (Adams et al., 1984, p. 1091). Flum (1994) suggests the addition to Marcia's classification of an evolutionary style that she believes can "reconcile the classic (turmoil) approach to adolescence and the empirical view (Coleman, 1978, 1980), which shows much less dramatic developmental change" (p. 497).

Religious affiliation, with regular attendance in Sunday School, confirmation, and Bar or Bat Mitzva in early adolescence, is followed by affiliations with religious organizations in late adolescence and young adulthood. These affiliations seem to facilitate a more solid identity process. Markstrom-Adams Hofstra, and Dougher (1994) found a connection between religion, church attendance, and identity formation. They studied Mormon and non-Mormon adolescents who were a minority nationally but were locally a majority. Mormons scored higher in identity foreclosure than Catholic or Protestant adolescents who were comparably a minority in the broader cultural sense, but were a majority in a narrower local sense. They suggest that "premature foreclosure among Mormon adolescents may be due to the importance of exhibiting indication of fidelity as efforts to strengthen one's minority identity and one's minority group in respect to the broader society . More frequent church attendance of Mormon adolescents was related to higher scores in commitment identity status (i.e., foreclosure and achievement)" (p. 453). For them, ego virtue is a "conceptual link between religion and identity formation" (p. 453). Fulton (1997) in his study of 257 college students at a Christian liberal arts college, came to the same conclusions. Erikson (1981) conceived of religious faith as a restoration of trust and hope arising in infancy and as the most lasting of institutional influences. The ego virtues of hope, will, purpose, and competence result from successful resolution of Erikson's first four psychosocial stages and are precursors of fidelity in adolescence. Fidelity acts as a "buffer against alienation by promoting belongingness through the use of rites, rituals, faith, and affirmative dogma" (p. 456).

Pollock (1983) viewed identity as being composed of various internal representations of the self, including social, economic, political, religious, professional, and scientific selves or identities. Different combinations of these selves in a progressive or regressive sense produce unique configurations of a person's personality, thus making possible various identities. Abend's (1974) scholarly paper constitutes a very serious effort to bring the concept into some relevant alignment with more modern ego psychology and concluded that *identity* is "a more limited concept, referring in fact to a specific part of the self" (p. 622). Many internal self representations, he says, are gathered together into a set of conscious and preconscious entities, whereas the *self* is a superordinate term encompassing a larger area of functioning of the personality.

Following Erikson, Abend's (1974) view is that:

> [Identity consists of] a loosely organized set of conscious and preconscious self-representations that serve to define the individual in a variety of social contexts. Included in its composition we would expect to find ideas regarding specific professional,

social, and sexual roles and preferences, aspects of the person's political and religious ideology and other unique values, and his more important personal interests and avocations. These self-representations are formed at a relatively high level of psychic development and are therefore complex products of instinctual drives, defenses, identifications, and sublimations, as well as reflecting the influence of these of constitutional givens and of the special contributions made by the particular individual's life experiences and opportunities [p. 620].

Abend goes on to say that an identity may have loose boundaries, but continuing development over a life span makes significant contributions to a changing identity, while at the same time possessing a self-sameness over time.

Kohut (1971) considered the concept *identity* too vague to be useful for modern psychoanalysis and proposed the terms *alter ego relationships* and *self–selfobject relationships* in the normative developmental context and also the merger transferences (twinship, grandiose, and idealized) in the pathological context. From a self psychological point of view a person's identity may refer to how a person is viewed by others, but more importantly to specifically unique aspects of the self. Kohut, in fact, insisted that identity did not belong in depth psychology, since it consisted of "observations of social behavior and the description of the (pre)conscious experience of oneself in the interaction with others" . . . (1971, pp. xiv–xv). To Erikson's credit, however, his descriptions clearly stipulate unconscious as well as conscious origins of identity and deserve to be considered part of a depth psychology. Muslin has expanded on Kohut's approach in his studies of the lives of Lyndon Johnson (Muslin, 1991), Gandhi (1995a), and Hitler (1995b). He weaves an extraordinarily rich psychological portrait of these individuals that is couched in self psychological language.

From this review it appears that psychoanalytic writers differ widely on the concept of and the seat for identity, some researchers insisting it is located in the self, while others locate it in the ego, the ego ideal, or the internal representational world. Still another view (as in the present work) would locate identity in a general sense within the whole character or personality, whether conscious or unconscious, and based on identifications and internalizations of affectively significant relationships. Erikson's answer to this debate is similar, in that a "pervasive sense of identity brings into gradual accord the variety of changing self-images that have been experienced during childhood (and that, during adolescence, can be dramatically recapitulated) and the role opportunities offering themselves to young people for selection and commitment" (p. 73).

The concept of identity has not enjoyed a firm foothold in any of the psychoanalytic schools of thought. From a classical theoretical perspective, identity is formed from the multiple identifications occurring from childhood onwards into adulthood and throughout the life cycle in terms of a construction of an integrated internal representational world (Sandler and Rosenblatt, 1962). Sandler and Rosenblatt correctly point out that the representational world is never an active agent, but is rather a set of guidelines (like a radar) by which the ego deploys appropriate defensive and adaptive operations. Loewald (1962) conceptualized this process as one by which "internalizations of relationships and interactions between the individual psychic apparatus and its environment are changed into inner relationships and interactions within the psychic apparatus" (p. 489). From an ego psychological point of view, identification processes are a form of internalization which results from separation–individuation strivings toward achieving autonomy. Identification processes occur mainly in connection with withdrawal of emotional investments in internal object relationships whether during resolution of the Oedipus complex, identification with an idealized figure, or mourning a real loss. In "Mourning and Melancholia," Freud (1917) conceived of the process of identification as following the abandonment of significant object cathexes. In metaphorical language, he said the "shadow" of the abandoned object "falls on the ego," which is transformed or altered by the taking in or introjection of the abandoned object. Bit by bit, identifications construct an identity. Identification with an aggressor, as a special form of identification, can and often is an important way of constructing an identity such as that of a dominating, controlling, and manipulative parent. Imitation often serves as an initial step in the identification process.

Schafer (1968) describes this process as the internalization of qualities and characteristics of another person: "all those processes by which the subject transforms real or imagined regulatory interactions with his environment, and real or imagined characteristics of his environment, into inner regulations and characteristics" (p. 9).

Conceptualization of *identity* is therefore best understood as a general concept of the entire personality or character. In fact, Meissner (1985) considers that the "notion of identity can be seen as providing an important bridge between the psychology of character and the psychology of the self" (p. 396). Identity is formed by all those internalizations and identifications with other persons who are valued and idealized but from whom the individual has achieved a certain enduring degree of separateness and autonomy. Identity is durable and stable in response to internal and external stressful pressures that threaten equilibrium. Identity includes social, emotional, political, religious, national, ethnic, and professional boundaries. In other words, identity is what a person is and does and becomes throughout the life cycle.

DEVELOPMENTAL CONSIDERATIONS

The problem for psychoanalysis is that while the term *identity* may be a global concept, it has major relevance in a clinical sense in young adulthood (Josselson, 1989). It combines under one rubric everything that constitutes a whole, integrated, and cohesive personality (or the superordinate self), including all those internalizations that make up the sexual, vocational, social, political, intellectual, and developmental parts of the personality. Identity formation in young adulthood is a process that normally takes place rather dramatically, even though beginning signs of identity formation appear early in life as part of the differentiation of the infant's personality in the mother–infant dyad. The ritualization of the mother–infant dyad is so skillfully choreographed by a mutual recognition that is at the same time so playful and formalized, evokes affects, and stimulates development in both affective and cognitive life. Emde's (1983, 1985, 1988) description of the "I-WE-GO" process in the toddler, and the emergence of an "I" as a crystallization of the executive functions in a personality, occurs out of a matrix of needs satisfactions over time. Throughout succeeding developmental stages, the continuing accretions are synthesized in a personality in the form of a definite identity. Erikson (1966, 1977) has described the various stages of ritualization in development which prove to be significant for positive or negative identity formation. The formalized and stereotyped rituals of recognition between mother and child are also highly individualized and exquisitely emotional in nature, including joy, surprise, and various degrees of pleasure and disapproval which enter into the construction of the first significant relationship (Stern, 1971, 1977, 1985). In the first six months, the infant becomes a "social being" and learns:

> How to invite his mother to play and then initiate an interaction with her; he will have become expert at maintaining and modulating the flow of social exchange; he will have acquired the signals to terminate or avoid an interpersonal encounter or just

place it temporarily in a "holding pattern." In general, he will have mastered most of the basic signals and conventions so that he can perform the "moves" and run off patterned sequences in step with those of his mother resulting in the dances that we recognize as social interactions. This biologically designed choreography will serve as a prototype for all his later interpersonal exchanges [Stern, 1977, p. 1].

All those efforts at seeking responsiveness from the significant caretakers are what the child observation researchers call "social referencing" (Sorce and Emde, 1981; Emde, 1983) and "refueling" (Speers, McFarland, Arnaud, and Curry, 1971). The differentiation of infants in the nursery one from another is relatively easy, even though occasionally caretakers have gotten babies' identities confused. This level of identity seems to be genetic and constitutional since certain unique and characteristic personality patterns are clearly and selectively limited to individuals. Constitutional factors were documented by Fries (1977), when she studied 200 neonates day and night from birth to the tenth day. Fries classified neonates into five groups in terms of their sensorimotor activity: "active, moderately active, and quiet, with extremes at each end—hyper and hypoactive" (p. 116). Follow-up studies showed that these groupings were sustained for thirty years! From infancy on, identity develops in increments through two general processes: identification and socialization. All these processes of interaction continue throughout the life cycle in a spiral of ever increasing complexity, and constitute very important components of the socialization process.

Young adults are subject to much pressure from peers and the culture in general in terms of the information explosion, the population explosion, and the threat of nuclear accidents, such as at Three Mile Island and Chernobyl. Young adults are disenchanted with a variety of institutional and political systems and values. The result is a turning away from intellectual interests, as in Bloom's pessimistic view (1987), even though I suspect that this extreme view is not entirely true since many people would attest to knowing young people who are actively and joyfully involved in intellectual pursuits. However, young adults are presented with a multitude of choices in terms of career as well as moral and ethical issues.

People who have resorted to a foreclosure of identity formation are familiar to us as bureaucratic personalities who exclude novelty and change from their lives, or those persons who fail to assimilate or integrate life's experiences and remain dilettantes. These are failures in the process of identity formation. This problem is not new since historians have noted pressures in modern Western cultures, and perhaps even greater ones in certain Eastern cultures, where the formlessness of life and "the onslaught of external events evoke inner formlessness and passivity; the diffuse identity becomes a technique of adjustment allowing one to cope with an incoherent, formless reality" (Stein and Vidich, 1960. p. 19). In fact, they say that democratic societies increase the range of possible identities, but interfere with the opportunity for the playful experimentation with various identities. Young medical students and resident physicians try out various identities as they move from one speciality service to another, temporarily identifying with the charismatic attending physicians who wear their stethoscopes around their necks, or on the neurology service place all the physical diagnostic tools in the breast pockets of their jackets or coats. The same playful experimentation occurs in other professions and in the trades as well. More recently, Adams et al. (1984) pointed out that if identity processes have not been initiated and integrated in late adolescence, individuals are more subject to peer and social pressures, and do not have sufficient adaptive capacities to make appropriate career choices. In fact, according to some recent research it appears that the development of higher level cognitive formal operations are important ingredients in identity formation (Klaczynski, Fauth, and Swanger, 1998). Job prospects become slimmer for those without a solid identity formation, and a bachelor's degree is not necessarily a sufficient guarantee of a good job, particularly in an era of downsizing when going to work for a major corporation can hardly be looked on as a lifetime career.

Currently, all over the world young people are turning to fundamentalist religions, cults, and "new age" religions for structure, family, and leadership in the acquisition of a purpose in life, ideals, values, and goals. Disillusionment with the overall erosion of morality in the culture or authoritarian government leadership, has led to mass suicides (e.g., the Jones Cult in Guyana, the Branch Davidians in Waco, Texas, and the Heaven's Gate group in San Diego, California).

SOCIALIZATION OF IDENTITY

Socialization processes involve resolution of multiple crises through decisions ranging from minor to major in the crucible within which identity formation emerges. The individual family and the level of family differentiation influences individuation, identity formation, and autonomy of each late adolescent and young adult. These influences, however, are discrete though indivisible phenomena. Individuation leads to greater autonomy that in turn facilitates more identity formation (Sabatelli and Mazon, 1985). As Marcia (1980) describes it, these "decisions are not made once and for all, but have to be made again and again. And the decisions may seem trivial at the time: whom to date, whether or not to break up, having intercourse, taking drugs, going to college or working, which college, what major, studying or playing, being politically active, and so on" (p. 161). Erikson (1966, 1977) described some of the ritualization experiences of adolescents and by inference young adults whereby young people are "enjoined to become responsible members of their society (or pseudo-species) and often of an elite within it" (1977, p. 107). There are those formal rites of confirmation, induction into elite groups, or graduation from school. Affiliative rituals involve instinctualized bonds with friends, lovers, and marriage partners. Marriage brings generational, parental, and didactic roles and responsibilities (Kaufman, 1971). Erikson said that ritualization "provides the psycho-social foundation for the gradual development of an independent identity to be sealed in adolescence by various rituals of confirmation, a second birth which will integrate all childhood identifications in a world view and belief system while making as ideologically foreign all those wishes and images which become undesirable." He uses the term *pseudo-speciation* which he defines as:

> [A] sense of irreversible difference between one's own and other kinds which can attach itself to evolved major differences among human populations or, indeed, to smaller and smallest differences which have come to loom large. In the form of man's "in" group loyalties, such a specific sense of being elite—as a tribe or nation, creed, class or ideology—can contribute to the highest achievements in citizenship, courage and workmanship and can, in fact, weld together in new loyalties (civis Romanus, Christian love) previously inimical entities. In the form of new "out" group enmities, on the other hand, it can express itself most variably in mortal hatred as well as in phobic avoidance, or in sheer clannishness. Such prejudice may make men more beastly than any beasts could be [such as the Nazi atrocities]; or it may, under peaceful conditions, make men vie with each other for the right vision or countervision within agreed-upon procedures [1977, pp. 76–77].

Members of an elite group or club differentiate themselves from others by joining together with common goals. Psychoanalytic institutes are no exception and may exhibit unique or special characteristics. One institute may promote the reputation of being very orthodox theoretically while another may promote the ideal of being open to questioning orthodoxy, while still others may adopt a research identity. Some groups may assume a specific identity, such as college fraternities that are distinguished by their scholastic interests, aims, and accomplishments while other college groups are known for having more social or athletic goals and values.

Turguet (1975) described the loss of personal identity in large groups such as the army, and in a most destructive fashion in a mob. There, the threat of anger leading to violence is very real. The loss of identity is experienced first as a fear of annihilation and the fear of the loss of one's boundaries (homogenation). Speaking loudly or being silent lowers the threshold for violence. The group demands action and the larger the group, the more the individual is frightened, and the group is detached from responsibility. One defense against these threats is institutionalization, promotion of leaders who create boundaries, and become more remote: then the leaders are idealized. Anger and criticism is projected onto the leader or a scapegoat is selected. What follows is a gradual and general breakdown of capacities for communication or listening to others. Projective mechanisms fail, and the natural tendency is to withdraw, thus creating more distress within the group.

From a sociological perspective, those civilizing processes that Freud discussed in *Civilization and Its Discontents* (1930) are lost, namely, the renunciation of instinctual gratifications and more centrally, the renunciation of infantile sexual claims on the oedipal object that lead to the cultural development of the individual. Work related and creative activities are derived from the civilizing influences of repression, sublimation, and disavowal of libidinal, narcissistic, and aggressive drives. These civilizing processes begin in the mother–infant dyad as formalized and ritualized (Erikson, 1966, 1977) but playfully evocative educational interactions of the mother with the emerging personality of the infant to encourage and stimulate the release of and modulating mastery over affects and bodily functions as well as the stimulation and development of unique skills and talents. A particular family's version of human existence assists its children in incorporating the culture of the larger society in increasingly complex rituals from infancy through adolescence into young adulthood. Developmental achievements in terms of the smiling response; the eighth-month anxiety experience; the acquisition of language; major and fine motor skills, and cognitive accretions are stimulated, destabilized, and resynthesized within the context of the dyadic processing relationship (Spitz, 1959). The experience of bonding (Kaufman, 1971), attachment (Bowlby, 1958), feeding, gratification, soothing, molding, and melding of the mother and infant in the primary relationship (Balint, 1949), or the symbiotic phase (Mahler, Pine, and Bergman, 1975), or the primitive self–selfobject relationship (Kohut, 1977), provides a foundation for the identification and socialization type of internalizations of the growing personality. Aronfreed (1969) discussed internalization in cognitive and affective terms, seeing cognitive aspects as being dependent on external reinforcement and conditioning processes of reward and punishment. The emotionally laden experiences of parenting stimulate the child's motivation for socialization and internalized controls.

These parental dyadic processes are carried forward into the formal settings of nursery school, kindergarten, secondary schools, college, and postgraduate programs where teachers, advisors, professors, classmates, and close friends play key roles in the shaping and consolidating of an identity. In the workplace, mentors in the professions of law and medicine as well as in the building or other trades produce the same results. Social referencing (Sorce and Emde, 1981) plays an important role in these processes throughout the life cycle. The role of the father in contributing to the formation of an identity has been studied by Cath (Cath, Gurwitt, and Gunsberg, 1989) and others, notably John Munder Ross (1984), Abelin (1971, 1975, 1980) and Herzog (1980).

Occupational choices (bricklayer, steel worker, writer, professional football player, doctor, lawyer, and opera singer) signify and contribute to identity formation (Laska and Micklin, 1979; Steinberg, Greenberger, Vaux, and Ruggiero, 1981). In fact, the process of professional socialization introduces very specific dimensions in the formation of identity structures or schemata. The law clerk, clinical internships, and residency programs, or apprentice programs for various trades provide on-the-job training for the learning and integration of practical knowledge with factual knowledge of a field. The professional socialization process adds a significant dimension to identity formation whereby the standards and values of the group shape and construct the identifications with group ideals. The learning of new skills, behavior patterns, and norms, values, and attitudes are internalized along with a new identity. Selection procedures and criteria limit admission to professional schools to those individuals whose qualifications compare favorably with those values, goals, ideals, and standards of a particular profession. Psychologically, these procedures increase motivation and commitment to the profession (Sabari, 1985). Professional socialization processes are heavily influenced by the emotions, fantasies, and psychodynamic processes of the student in a professional school (Levinson, 1967). "Career failure becomes the major disaster to those who commit their total selves to a job . . . work identities have been invested with profound meaning . . ."; "The job becomes the main basis for self-justification" (Stein and Vidich, 1960, p. 25). Failures to achieve advancement in careers, such as making partner in a law firm or failing to advance in a specialty training program result in a severe and persistent narcissistic injury. Stein and

Vidich (1960) advocate a kind of loosening of a rigid identity so that a playfulness ensues that leads to different identities being tried in a mass society so riddled with conflicting pressures; for example, college and graduate students may identify with different professors every quarter or change political views or religious affiliation. Also, young actors must be able to shift roles so as to not become rigidly typecast.

Postgraduate or postdoctoral education, such as in the psychoanalytic training programs, prepare the young adult candidate to be technically skillful and personally qualified. Even though candidates may be in their middle or even late thirties, their emotional development has been delayed because of lengthy college and professional school training programs. In fact, Wells (1989) found "many medical students are developmentally at an adolescent level, and many who are striving to become young adults are encouraged by the nature of the medical school experience itself to remain immersed in adolescent issues" (p. 228). There is much that is involved in the socialization process, however, that is obtained in the relationship with the training analyst, the supervisors, and the classroom instructors. The latter's devotion to the ideal of an unswerving search for the truth facilitates the internalization of such psychoanalytic values in a receptive candidate who has benefited from a good analytic experience. The expanding internal qualities of a psychoanalytic identity involve, according to Dewald (1987), unconscious processes in the context of a subculture of candidate, supervisor, and training analyst. Various loyalties and identifications with the candidate's analyst, supervisor, and favorite teachers (all of whom are role models), have unconscious transference meanings in terms of hopes of fulfillment of unconscious grandiose infantile and childhood fantasies. Integration of these identifications (Joseph and Widlocher, 1983), and professional role models, normally takes place in the latter part of the training program, but proceeds throughout the analyst's professional life (L. Grinberg, 1983). Klauber (1983) asserted that the psychoanalyst undergoes a process of conversion of "mind and heart" through many kinds of analytic experiences that he calls a "metanoia." He went on to indicate that the psychoanalyst must have an analytic fire in his belly to learn the field and practice the profession. Then over a long period of time the psychoanalyst's identity gradually consolidates, or under some specific pressures it may undergo regression and disintegration (L. Grinberg and R. Grinberg, 1971, 1974).

Kernberg especially referred to superego and ego ideal functioning of candidates in terms of a "firmness of convictions moderated by a degree of flexibility of value systems" (1987b, p. 64). The psychoanalytic identity of graduate analysts and candidates alike is taken up in great depth by Chasseguet-Smirgel (1987). The social, economic, and political pressures that influence, erode, and otherwise modify the psychoanalytic identity of the younger analysts are serious issues that are operating today over a decade later, and are in fact even more serious than was the case in 1987. One extremely serious pressure has been the advent of managed care prepayment plans and HMOs that have eroded the patient population, restricted the length of therapy, and effectively limited patients' access to expert care. Young graduates of psychology and social work training programs face these same reality issues that make entry into their professional field extremely difficult.

Group pressures can pose a severe threat to the personal identity of individuals when they are forced to choose between their own values instead of giving in to conventionality and social pressures within an institute. Unanalyzed, narcissistic self-serving needs emerge from an immature ego ideal and a sadistic superego that demands perfection and has unrealistic expectations of others. Sometimes these issues are not revealed until the candidate is in supervision when, for example, he sees only his own dynamics in his patients, lacks curiosity, searches out professional alternatives, becomes bored with the field, or demands a rigid doctrinaire position. Arrogant struggles for power within institutes often seem to be derived from unresolved and unanalyzed narcissistic problems. These struggles for power occur in those individuals whose development has been delayed because of the lengthy training programs, so that even though they are in their middle thirties, they behave as if they are late adolescent or young adults (Wells, 1989). Proselytizing of younger colleagues to create a following is an ominous factor in this regard too.

However, a core identity of the psychoanalyst is derived from a successful psychoanalytic exploration of his own unconscious, leading to a discovery of unconscious meanings and the reality of unconscious determinism. The acquisition of an enduring, authentic insight combined with a solid cognitive and emotional awareness for one's neurotic conflicts that are thoroughly worked through, realistic concern for oneself, and empathic humanistic concern for one's patients, are all part of the core identity of a psychoanalyst. Self-analysis, too, assists in maintaining this identity.

CLINICAL EXAMPLE

A 25-year-old single woman who had recently graduated from college returned home when her attempts to find a satisfying career and a suitable heterosexual partner had resulted in repeated failures. She was devastated from both these endeavors, but she was mostly humiliated by the return to her family's home, feeling she had been forced back into a child's role. She had been living a relatively self-sufficient and more or less self-sustaining life in everyday decision making. But upon returning home she felt she didn't know what to do with herself or what course of action to take. She was virtually paralyzed and demoralized. Finally, she obtained a clerical job in a large office. When she presented herself for therapy, she was most unhappy and bewildered. In fact, she said she had always been unhappy as far back as she could remember. Despite a certain waiflike bewilderment, however, there was a certain proud self-contained quality that suggested an unrealized, untapped inner strength. Depressive affect was accompanied by a listlessness and a moderate sleep disturbance. Bored with her various low level and mentally unchallenging jobs, she looked for an opportunity to make a change, but when opportunities for occupational change were presented to her, she realized the problem was more an internal one and knew she had to address the reasons for her inner affective life. She had also withdrawn from all friends, fearing that she would have to explain what was going on inside, and that she felt she had nothing to say anyway. Everyone else seemed so happy or able to cope with life's frustrations, and it puzzled her that no one seemed to understand what she was experiencing. She found it hard to believe that I, as her therapist, could possibly appreciate her predicament.

In a short time, when a reasonably strong alliance had been established, she was able to open up enough to reveal a number of issues of long standing that had given rise to helplessness, and suppressed and repressed anger. As the reasons that provoked her angry emotions were revealed, she began to feel less helpless and depressed. The loss of identity and identity diffusion issues remained to be addressed, but the beginning phase of treatment gave her courage to speak out about various injustices she felt she had experienced as she was growing up. Signs of a beginning solid inner core self emerged and the coalescing of a cohesive identity soon followed.

Family disputes interfere with identity formation and delay the developmental process of identity formation predominately when there is less cohesion within the family, psychological distress within individual family members, and deviant behavior (Fondacaro, Dunkle, and Pathak, 1998).

FREUD'S IDENTITY

Over the past few years, there has been a great deal of interest in the psychobiographical study of Freud's personality and his identity. Trosman (1985) has constructed Freud's identity as a Jew, an expert clinician, a serious scientist, and an intellectual with far-ranging interests. In the course of his work, Trosman sees Freud as having an avowed Jewish identity, which was fiercely humanitarian. While he was a political revolutionary in adolescence, Freud abandoned that identity as a young adult and his personality evolved into that of a scientific revolutionary as he founded the new field of psychoanalysis. His identity was composed of a basic Jewishness, but as Trosman so thoroughly documents, Freud's identity was heavily influenced by his teachers in the gymnasium and the university: Brucke, the scientist, Brentano (philosopher and ex-priest), and Meynert, professor of psychiatry at the University of Vienna. Charcot, the famous French neurologist and founder of a school of hypnosis, and Joseph Breuer, a prominent internist and collaborator with Freud, were later but equally important influences. Freud was exposed to all these teachers who had broad cultural interests and had received classical educations. His own education was so thorough that at one point he confidently volunteered to translate John Stuart Mill's work for one of his teachers (Gomperz). Greek, Roman, and ancient Egyptian cultures captured his imagination, while literary interests of a wide scope, including Dickens, Shakespeare, Heine, and Goethe, enriched his writing style. Brentano was a favorite teacher at the university, and Freud took many courses from him in philosophy. On more than one occasion he "proved" the existence of God to a point where Freud was unable to mount a successful rebuttal. Freud experienced some Teutonic tugs (Trosman, 1985, p. 21) during World War I when he identified with the cause of the Central Powers, but he did not join in with the Austrian identification with German Nationalism preceding World War II.

In World War I, Freud was obviously torn, because three of his sons served in the Austrian army, two of whom saw a great deal of action. His son Martin was wounded and a son-in-law, Sophie's husband, was wounded and discharged. Several of his colleagues also served (Eitingon, Ferenczi, Abraham, and Rank). Peter Gay (1988) notes that "The needs of psychoanalysis, like the news from his sons at the front, tested the limits of Freud's patriotism" (p. 351). On the other hand, Gay remarks that Freud "continued to identify the cause of the Central Powers as his own, and was irritated by Jones's unfailing confidence in the victory of the Allies" (p. 353). He was so appalled by the bloody carnage on both sides that he wrote "Thoughts for the Times on War and Death" (1915).

Instead, Trosman (1985, p. 83) persuasively argues that Freud identified more strongly with literary figures in his self-analysis. While resonating with the implied unconscious wishes of Hamlet and Oedipus, consolidation of Freud's identity was taking place through the process of finding a solution to his now conscious oedipal wishes. Freud's personality comes credibly to life in Trosman's thesis. It is a tightly woven and highly reasoned but essentially psychoanalytic exposition of the known and not so well-known facts about Freud's life, personality development, and especially the emergence and flowering of his intellectual, literary, artistic, and linguistic skills; in short, his identity and his genius. Freud (1941) shared in the ethical and humanitarian interests and values of the Jewish organization B'nai B'rith, and he was very identified with his Jewish heritage. In a presentation to that group he said he valued his own Jewish identity when he referred to his freedom to use his intellect and "do without agreement with the compact majority" (p. 274). There was within him what he considered to be a very powerful drive almost indescribable in words which connected up with a "clear consciousness of an inner identity, the safe privacy of a common mental construction" (p. 274). Robert (1976) constructs an attractive though somewhat romanticized thesis that Freud's identity grew out of a special Jewish mind-set that differentiated him from Gentiles (i.e., an "essential Jewishness"), expanding contact with his rich inner emotional life and his assimilation of the best in classical Western education and culture. Freud's passion for political revolutionary ideas as an adolescent grew into a scientific revolution as he created psychoanalysis with his dream book.

> Freud lived on terms of natural intimacy with the great figures of the Bible, they were so much a part of his inner life that he felt himself to be in turns Joseph, Jacob, and Moses—Joseph because he too was an expert in the interpretation of dreams; Jacob, because in his old age his children took him, too, to Egypt [England]; and Moses, because, in fighting for a "temporal conception of life and the conquest of magic thought, the rejection of mysticism," which according to him were the true message of Moses, he was in his own way continuing the lawgiver's work of liberation [Robert, 1976, p. 37].

Shengold's (1971) scholarly elaboration of Freud's identification with the Biblical Joseph is clearly spelled out. He made the connection of himself as the patriarch Jacob leaving his homeland to escape to the refuge of England (Egypt). Also, the liberal Austrian Emperor Joseph was very important to the Freud family since he decreed that Jews should have civil rights and be eligible to serve in the military. This stimulated the young Sigmund to have phantasies about becoming a military hero like the Semitic General Hannibal. In fact, Freud had three "favorite heroes—Hannibal; Marcus Brutus, the defender of the Roman Republic; and Karl Moor, the protagonist of Schiller's *The Robbers*—all shared a passionate dedication to freedom in the face of tyranny. Freud's deep and lasting interest in them points up his own political sympathies and has an important bearing on his later intellectual and emotional development" (McGrath, 1986, pp. 59–60). McGrath also emphasized the importance of the newly bound Phillipson Bible that Jakob Freud gave to his son on his thirty-fifth birthday.

Peter Gay (1987, 1988) has written eloquently about Freud and religion or rather his antireligious interests. Gay, in fact, documents Freud's avowed atheistic position. Yerushalmi (1991), however, makes a very credible case for why Freud obscured his Jewishness, his familiarity with Hebrew and Yiddish, as well as Judaism. Jakob Freud had wanted to assimilate into the dominant Viennese culture and disavow his Galician family past. Soon after arriving in Vienna, he "dispensed with the Jewish dietary observations and with most of the customary rituals; with the only exception I know of was the festival meal of Seder on the eve of Passover" (Jones, 1957, pp. 350–351). But beginning at age seven Freud grew up reading the famous Phillipson Bible with its 500 woodcuts and intellectual commentary on early history and comparative religion. Yiddish was his mother's primary language and he could well have grown up speaking with her in that emotionally rich and folkwise language. In central Europe, Yiddish was a universal language which made it easy for travelers to communicate with each other. To further buttress his case, Yerushalmi points out that Jakob Freud gave his son Sigmund on his thirty-fifth birthday the famous Philipson family Bible (Ostow, 1989) and inscribed in it his favorite verses in Hebrew. Furthermore, Yerushalmi asserts that Freud was so steeped in a Jewish identity, even if he did renounce Judaism as a religion, that he could not escape the fact he was deeply committed to being a Jew. E. Rice (1992) makes the same argument in a letter to *The Forward*. Rice (1990) refers to a visit Theodore Reik paid to Freud's mother and was impressed that she spoke only a Galician Yiddish. Henry Bondi, whose parents, grandparents, and great-grandparents were lifelong friends of the family of Martha Bernays Freud, going back to Martha's grandfather, Rabbi Isaac Bernays, who was chief rabbi of Hamburg (Orthodox) from 1821 to 1849, makes the same point, according to Rice. Most eastern European Jews, especially the upwardly mobile and educated ones, who migrated westward to Germany and Austria, Rice says, were determined to divest themselves of their Galician past, including Yiddish. But neither Amalia nor Jakob had any formal education. Even though Freud denied that he spoke or wrote in that language, his mother spoke only Yiddish, so it is safe to conclude Freud *must have been very fluent* in Yiddish at least during his childhood. McGrath's (1986) constructions point out that Freud's nephew and playmate John was the model for all of Freud's future brotherly relationships—the loved and hated friend and rival, who was often combined in the same individual. Freud was steeped in the fact that one of the essences of being a Jew is abiding by the Commandments (Owen, 1987) and all their implied meanings. Furthermore, Rice (1990) also documents that the Austrian government mandated that all boys and girls of the Jewish community had to study Hebrew from the age of 7 to the age of 18. Since Freud was at the top of his class every year, he surely must have retained some knowledge of the Hebrew language well into adulthood.

SUMMARY

Identity development is probably the central esssential developmental task of the young adult. This achievement certainly begins in early childhood and proceeds through later child-hood, while noting body changes and differences of the sexes. Curiosity about the origin of babies and the early interests of sexuality participate in the process of identity formation. Ado-lescent intellectual interests and socialization add further di-mensions to the process. But in the young adult, a powerful and massive contribution takes place in the reshaping and re-configuration of this developmental achievement.

Marcia's (1980) four types of identity formation include identity achievement, foreclosure, identity diffusion, and mor-atorium that are defined by the presence or absence of a crisis and commitment to a vocation and an ideology. Marcia sup-ports and expands on Erikson's views of identity formation. Various studies indicate that religious affiliation and education facilitate identity formation in many young people.

The views expressed here are that identity formation can best be understood as a general theory of the personality as a whole bridging the space between concepts of character and self whether the self is thought to be a subordinate or superor-dinate structure. Internalization of specific and unique quali-ties and characteristics are inculcated into the personality including social, emotional, political, religious, national, eth-nic, and professional boundaries.

REFERENCES

Abelin, E. L. (1971), The role of the father in the separation–individuation process. In: *Separation-Individuation,* ed. J. B. McDevitt & C. F. Settlage. New York: International Universities Press.

————— (1975), Some further observations and comments on the earliest role of the father. *Internat. J. Psycho-Anal.,* 56:293–302.

————— (1980), Triangulation, the role of the father and the origins of core identity during the rapprochement subphase, In: *Rapprochement: The Critical Subphase of Separation Individuation,* ed. R. F. Lax, S. Bach, & J. A. Burland. New York: Jason Aronson, pp. 151–169.

Abend, S. M. (1974), Problems of identity, theoretical and clinical applica-tions. *Psychoanal. Quart.,* 43:606–637.

Adams, G. R., Ryan, J. H., Hoffman, J. J., Dobson, W. R., & Nielsen, E. C. (1984), Ego identity status, conformity behavior, and personality in late adolescence. *J. Personal. & Soc. Psychology*, 47:1091–1110.

Aronfreed, J. (1969), The concept of internalization. In: *Handbook of Socialization Theory and Research*, ed. D. A. Goslin. Chicago: Rand-McNally.

Balint, M. (1949), Early developmental states of the ego: Primary object love. *Internat. J. Psycho-Anal.*, 30:265–273.

Bernstein, H. (1963), Identity and sense of identity. Paper presented at the Chicago Psychoanalytic Society, February 26.

Bloom, A. (1987), *The Closing of the American Mind*. New York: Simon & Schuster.

Bowlby, J. (1958), The nature of the child's tie to his mother. *Internat. J. Psycho-Anal.*, 39:350–373.

Cath, S., Gurwitt, A., & Gunsberg, L. (1989), *Fathers and Their Families*. Hillside, NJ: Analytic Press.

Chasseguet-Smirgel, J., Ed.(1987), *Maintenance of the Psychoanalytic Identity and Functioning in a World of Flux*, Monogr. 6. London: International Psychoanalytic Association.

Coleman, C. F. (1978), Current contradictions in adolescent theory. *J. Youth Adol.*, 7:1–12.

——— (1980), *The Nature of Adolescence*. London: Methuen.

Dewald, P. (1987), *Learning Process in Psychoanalytic Supervision: Complexities and Challenges*. Madison, CT: International Universities Press.

Emde, R. (1983), The pre-representational self and its affective core. *The Psychoanalytic Study of the Child*, 38:165–192. New Haven, CT: Yale University Press.

——— (1985), Emotional availability, shared meaning, and the origins of the "We-go." Paper presented at Chicago Psychoanalytic Society, June 25.

——— (1988), Development terminable and interminable. 1. Innate and motivational factors from infancy. *Internat. J. Psycho-Anal.*, 69:23–42.

Erikson, E. H. (1956), The problem of ego identity. *J. Amer. Psychoanal. Assn.*, 4:56–121.

——— (1959), Identity and the Life Cycle. *Psychological Issues*, Monogr. 1. New York: International Universities Press.

——— (1966), Ontogeny of ritualization. In: *Psychoanalysis—A General Psychology: Essays in Honor of Heinz Hartmann*, ed. R. M. Loewenstein, L. M. Newman, M. Schur, & A. J. Solnit. New York: International Universities Press, pp. 601–621.

——— (1977), *Toys and Reasons—Stages in the Ritualization of Experience*. New York: W. W. Norton.

——— (1981), The Galilean Sayings and the sense of "I." *Yale Rev.*, 70:321–362.

——— (1982), *The Life Cycle Completed*. New York: W. W. Norton.

Flum, H. (1994), The evolutive style of identity formation. *J. Youth & Adol.,* 23:489–498.

Fondacaro, M. R., Dunkle, M. E., & Pathak, M. K. (1998), Procedural justice in resolving family disputes, a psychosocial analysis of individual and family functioning in late adolescence. *J. Youth & Adol.,* 27:101–119.

Freud, S. (1915), Thoughts for the times on war and death. *Standard Edition,* 14:273–300. London: Hogarth Press, 1957.

———— (1917), Mourning and melancholia. *Standard Edition,* 14:237–258. London: Hogarth Press, 1957.

———— (1930), Civilization and Its Discontents. *Standard Edition,* 21:57–145. London: Hogarth Press, 1961.

———— (1941), Address to the Society of B'nai B'rith. *Standard Edition,* 20:271–274. London: Hogarth Press, 1959.

Fries, M. E. (1977), Longitudinal study: Pregenital period to parenthood. *J. Amer. Psychoanal. Assn.,* 25:115–132.

Fulton, A. S. (1997), Identity status, religious orientation, and prejudice. *J. Youth & Adol.,* 26:1–11.

Gay, P. (1987), *A Godless Jew.* New Haven, CT: Yale University Press.

———— (1988), *Freud: A Life for Our Time.* New York: W. W. Norton.

Gray, S. H. (1990), Developmental issues in young adulthood: Psychoanalytic perspectives. *Adol. Psychiatry,* 17:328–337.

Grinberg, L. (1983), Discussion. In: *The Identity of the Psychoanalyst,* ed. E. Joseph & D. Widlocher. Monogr., 2:51–66. International Psycho-Analytic Association.

———— Grinberg, R. (1966), The acquisition of the sense of identity in the psychoanalytic process, tr. P. Brockman. *Rev. Psychoanal.* (Uruguay), 8:247–254.

———— ———— (1971), *Identidad y Cambio.* Buenos Aries: Kargieman.

———— ———— (1974), The problem of identity and the psychoanalytic process. *Internat. Rev. Psychoanal.,* 1:499–507.

Herzog, J. (1980), Sleep disturbance and father hunger in 18–28-month-old boys: The Erlkonig Syndrome. *The Psychoanalytic Study of the Child,* 35: 219–233. New Haven, CT: Yale University Press.

Holland, N. (1985), *The I.* New Haven, CT: Yale University Press.

Jacobson, E. (1964), *The Self and the Object World.* New York: International Universities Press.

Jones, E. (1957), *The Life and Work of Sigmund Freud,* Vol. 3. New York: Basic Books.

Joseph, E., & Widlocher, D. Eds., (1983), *The Identity of the Psychoanalyst.* IPA Monogr. 2. New York: International Universities Press.

Josselson, R. (1989), Identity formation in adolescence: Implications for young adulthood. In: *Adolescent Psychiatry,* 16:142–154. Chicago: University of Chicago Press.

Kaufman, I. C. (1971), Biologic considerations of parenthood. In: *Parenthood: Its Psychology and Psychopathology*, ed. E. J. Anthony & T. Benedek. Boston: Little, Brown, pp. 3–55.

Kernberg, O. (1980), *Internal World and External Reality*. New York: Jason Aronson.

———— (1987a), Restructuring the superego and the ego ideal. *J. Amer. Psychoanal. Assn.*, 36:1005–1029.

———— (1987b), The basic intrapsychic organization of the analyst and the features which threaten or favor the maintenance of the psychoanalytic identity and functioning. In: *Maintenance of the Psychoanalytic Identity and Functioning in a World in Flux*, IPA Monograph 6, ed. J. Chasseguet-Smirgel. London: International Psychoanalytic Association, pp. 63–76.

Klaczynski, P. A., Fauth, J. M., & Swanger, A. (1998), Adolescent identity: Rational vs. experiential processing, formal operations, and clinical thinking beliefs. *J. Youth & Adol.*, 27:185–207.

Klauber, J. (1983), The identity of the psychoanalyst. In: *The Identity of the Psychoanalyst*, IPA Monogr. 2, ed. E. D. Joseph, & D. Widlocher. New York: International Universities Press, pp. 41–50.

Kohut, H. (1971), *The Analysis of the Self*. New York: International Universities Press.

———— (1977), *The Restoration of the Self*. New York: International Universities Press.

Kramer, P. (1955), On discovering one's identity. A case report. *The Psychoanalytic Study of the Child*, 10:47–74. New York: International Universities Press.

Laska, S. B., & Micklin, M. (1979), The knowledge dimension of occupational socialization. Role models and their social influence. *Youth & Soc.*, 10:360–378.

Levinson, D. (1967), Medical education and the theory of adult socialization. *J. Health & Soc. Behav.*, 8:253–265.

Loewald, L. (1962), Internalization, separation, mourning, and the superego. *Psychoanal. Quart.*, 31:483–504.

Mahler, M. S., Pine, F., & Bergman, A. (1975), *The Psychological Birth of The Human Infant*. New York: Basic Books.

Marcia, J. E. (1980), Identity in adolescence. In: *Handbook of Adolescent Psychology*, ed. J. Adelson. New York: Wiley, pp.159–187.

Markstrom-Adams, C., Hofstra, G., & Dougher, K. (1994), The ego-virtue of fidelity: A case for the study of religion and identity formation in adolescence. *J. Youth & Adol.*, 23:453–469.

McGrath, W. J. (1986), *Freud's Discovery of Psychoanalysis: The Politics of Hysteria*. Ithaca, NY: Cornell University Press.

Meissner, W. W. (1985), Theories of personality and psychopathology: Classical psychoanalysis. In: *Comprehensive Textbook of Psychiatry*, Vol. 1, ed. H. I. Kaplan & B. J. Sadock. Baltimore: Williams & Wilkins, pp. 347–348.

Muslin, H., *Lyndon Johnson: The Tragic Self. A Psychoanalytic Portrait.* New York: Plenum Press.

—— (1995a), Ghandi. Typescript.

—— (1995b), Hitler. Typescript.

Offer, D., & Offer, J. B. (1975), *From Teenage to Young Manhood.* New York: Basic Books.

Ostow, M. (1989), Sigmund Freud and the Phillipson Bible. *Internat. Rev. Psychoanal.* 16:483–492.

Owen, R. (1987), On becoming a Jew. *Commentary,* 84:55–62.

Oxford Dictionary, Compact Edition. (1971), s.v. "Identity."

Panel (1958), Problems of identity. Reporter D. Rubinfine. *J. Amer. Psychoanal. Assn.,* 6:612–627.

Pollock, G. H. (1983), Self and identity: The psychoanalyst, psychoanalysis and society. In: *The Identity of the Psychoanalyst,* ed. E. Joseph & D. Widlocher. New York: International Universities Press, pp. 195–206.

Rapaport, D., & Gill, M. (1959), The points of view and assumptions of metapsychology. *Internat. J. Psycho-Anal.,* 40:153–162.

Rice, E. (1990), *Freud and Moses.* Albany, NY: State University of New York Press.

—— (1992), Letters to the Editor, Sigmund Freud and Yiddish. *The Forward.* March 6, p. 7.

Robert, M. (1976), *From Oedipus to Moses,* tr. R. Manheim. Garden City, N Y: Anchor Press/Doubleday.

Ross, J. M. (1984), The darker side of fatherhood: Clinical and developmental ramifications of the "Laius Motif." In: *The Oedipus Papers,* ed. G. P. Pollock & J. M. Ross. New York: International Universities Press, pp. 389–417.

Sabari, J. S. (1985), Professional socialization: Implications for occupational therapy education, *J. Amer. Occup. Ther.,* 39:96–102.

Sabatelli, R. M., & Mazon, A. (1985), Differentiation, individuation, and identity formation: The integration of family system and individual developmental perspectives. *Adolescence,* 20:619–633.

Sandler, J., & Rosenblatt, B. (1962), The concept of the representational world. *The Psychoanalytic Study of the Child,* 17:128–145. New York: International Universities Press.

Schafer, R. (1968), *Aspects of Internalization.* New York: International Universities Press.

Shengold, L. (1971), Freud and Joseph. In: *The Unconscious Today. Essays in Honor of Max Schur.* New York: International Universities Press, pp. 473–484.

—— (1980), More on rats and rat people. In: *Freud and His Patients,* Vol. 2, ed. M. Kanzer & J. Glenn. New York: Jason Aronson, pp. 180–202.

Sorce, J. F., & Emde, R. N. (1981), Mother's presence is not enough. *Develop. Psychol.,* 17:737–745.

Speers, R. W., McFarland, M. B., Arnaud, S. H., & Curry, N. E. (1971), Recapitulation of separation-individuation processes when the normal three-year-old enters nursery school. In: *Separation Individuation,* ed. J. B. McDevitt & C. F. Settlage. New York: International Universities Press, pp. 297–321.

Spitz, R. (1959), *A Genetic Field Theory of Ego Formation.* New York: International Universities Press.

Stein, M. R., & Vidich, A. J. (1960), Identity and history. In: *Identity and Anxiety,* ed. M. R. Stein, A. J. Vidich, & D. M. White. Glencoe, IL: Free Press, pp. 17–33.

Steinberg, L. D., Greenberger, E., Vaux, A., & Ruggiero, M. (1981), Early work experience: Effects on adolescent occupational socialization. *Youth & Soc.,* 12:403–422.

Stern, D. (1971), A micro-analysis of mother–infant interaction: Behaviors regulating social contact between a mother and her three-and-a-half-month-old twins. *J. Amer. Acad. Child Psychiatry,* 10:501–517.

———— (1977), *The First Relationship: Infant and Mother.* Cambridge, MA.: Harvard University Press.

———— (1985), *The Interpersonal World of the Infant.* New York: Basic Books.

Tausk, V. (1919), On the origins of the "influencing machine." In: *The Psychoanalytic Reader,* ed. R. Fleiss. New York: International Universities Press, 1948, pp. 52–85.

Trosman, H. (1985), *Freud and the Imaginative World.* Hillsdale, NJ: Analytic Press.

Turguet, P. (1975), The large group. In: *The Large Group: Dynamics and Therapy,* ed. L. Kreeger. London: Constable, pp. 87–144.

Wells, L. A. (1989), Common issues of late adolescence and young adulthood in medical students. *Adol. Psychiatry,* 16:228–245. Chicago: University of Chicago Press.

Wertsch, J. V. (1985), *Vygotsky and the Socialization of Mind.* Cambridge, MA: Harvard University Press.

Wheelis, A. (1958), *The Quest for Identity.* New York: W. W. Norton.

———— (1959), Psychoanalysis and identity. *Psychoanal. Rev.,* 46:65–74.

Yerushalmi, Y. H. (1991), *Freud's Moses: Judaism Terminable and Interminable.* New Haven, CT: Yale University Press.

Chapter 3

Gender and Sexual Identity

The terms *gender identity* and *sexual identity* in the psychoanalytic literature are confusing at best, but the definitions in Money and Ehrhardt's (1972) classic book *Man and Woman Boy and Girl* are helpful and elegant in their simplicity. They speak of psychosexual *differentiation* beginning with the prenatal period of embryonic development and continuing throughout the postnatal period of social and psychological development. They emphasize the theme of a complex interaction of hormones, chromosomes, genes, and environmental influences. Their emphasis on their experience with hermaphrodites and pseudohermaphrodites, and the presence of a suitable penis to guide them in making decisions about sex reassignment, has been seriously questioned by Diamond and Sigmundson's (1997) long-term review of the case of a boy as well as by an editorial (Reiner, 1997). *Gender identity* is defined by Money and Ehrhardt "as the sameness, unity, and persistence of one's individuality as male or female (or ambivalent) in greater or lesser degree, especially as it is experienced in self awareness of behavior. Gender identity is the private experience of gender role and gender role is the public expression of gender identity" (p. 284). In Zucker and Bradley's (1995) experience, gender identity is taken very seriously by preschoolers in their affective responses to questions if they belong to the opposite sex. Gender disorders in children, usually males, often lead to adolescent and young adult homosexuality. In special cases, psychoanalytic therapeutic intervention can felicitously transform this trajectory from a gay orientation into a solid heterosexual one (Greenson, 1966; Haber, 1991). Most researchers in this area, including Tyson (1998), use a model consisting of gender identity, gender role, and sexual orientation. Gender role refers to "behaviors, attitudes, and personality traits that a society, in a given culture and historical period, designates as masculine or feminine social role" (Zucker and Bradley, 1995, p. 3). This includes in young children same-sex versus opposite-sex affiliative preference behavior, "fantasy roles, toy interests, dress-up play, and interest in rough-and-tumble play" (Zucker and Bradley, 1995, p. 3). Sexual orientation refers to how a person responds to sexual stimuli.

Disorders in gender identity formation occur in many forms, including the perversions, transsexuality, and fetishistic behavior (Coates, Friedman, and Wolf, 1991). Gender identity disorders can be seen as compromise formations of multiple factors, but patterns of sexuality, whether heterosexual or homosexual, must be understood in a very complex matrix of biological, sociological, and psychological influences. Haber (1991) described a case of a 3 years, 9 months old boy who wished he was a girl; he cross-dressed, played with dolls, and pretended he was a superheroine. Psychoanalysis uncovered a feminine identification defense against hierarchically organized fears of "loss of the object, anal loss, and castration by the object reorganized in all libidinal phases through latency" (p. 107). A previous report by Greenson (1966), of a $5^{1}/_{2}$-year-old boy who had started cross-dressing two years earlier, revealed a similar defensive identification with a powerful mother who was simultaneously being analyzed by Stoller. "She wished the marked femininity on her son and he had complied without any observable struggle before he was a year old" (Stoller, 1985, p. 394).

The father was a business failure and a weak person who was rarely at home. The parents rarely had sex and when they quarreled, father went home to his mother. The mother was proud of her son as though he were her possession. Greenson (1968) proposed the concept of "disidentifying" with mother in the process of separation-individuation, which was incomplete in the case of the boy described in the 1966 paper. Earlier, Greenson (1964) described an unusual case of a World War II paratrooper who changed his gender, surgically altering his body to conform to a "circumscribed, well-organized delusional system" (p. 218) since he firmly believed he must be a woman when he fell in love with a man, being unable to admit to homosexual feelings. An even more curious case of a transsexual was that of a young man who succeeded in persuading the surgeons to change his gender. He then had a lesbian relationship with his former girl friend. Bettelheim (1954) used anthropological and psychoanalytic observations to address the complex psychological interests of children who wish to be the opposite sex and possess the genitals of the other gender. Males envy the woman's power and the strength they perceive in the woman's capacity to bear children, her breasts, and the ability to nurse her children, while females envy the man's penis and his superior muscular power.

GENDER IDENTITY

Kleeman (1972) was a pioneer in calling attention to the fact that Freud's theoretical formulations lacked a discussion of gender identity in male (1965), *and* in female sexual development (1966) as well, since in Freud's day neurohormonal and genetic information had not been discovered. One of the most outstanding contributions in this area was the seminal work of Money and Ehrhardt (1972) and Robert Stoller (1966, 1968a,b,

1985). Both of these research studies of those "natural experiments" in primarily biologically based and subsequent psychological aberrations in gender and sexual identity, led them to suggest that "masculinity or femininity is defined here as any quality that is felt by its possessor to be masculine or feminine . . . a belief—more precisely a dense mass of beliefs, . . . and not an incontrovertible fact" (Stoller, 1985, p. 11). Stoller goes on to outline what he considers to be core gender identity which is firmly set in place by the age of 2 or 3 years. His five points may be summarized as follows:

1. A biologically or physiologically based organization of the fetal brain through the presence of certain specific hormones. For example, testosterone is converted into estrogen in certain concentrations in the undifferentiated fetus brain to transform it into a male brain. This is extrapolated from work done on lower mammals (MacLusky and Naftolin, 1981).
2. Assignment of sex by the attending physicians and parents.
3. Parental attitudes, especially that of mothers, of their infant's sex and each infant's organization of these perceptions into a hierarchy of motivations.
4. Certain ways of handling infants, that is, conditioning, imprinting, or other forms of learning, which Stoller calls "biopsychic phenomena" and which he speculates "permanently modify the infant's brain and behavior" (1985, p. 12).
5. The organization in the brain of sensations from the entire body and especially the genitalia, that constitute the body image (Schilder, 1938) and correspond to the body-ego (Freud, 1923) or the body-self (Kohut, 1971).

These five factors operate in the overall development of gender identity. It is clear, therefore, if one accepts Stoller's formulations, that gender identity is a very complex process involving structures which are derived from biological, psychological, and caretaking influences. In his 1968 book, Stoller emphasized the importance of cultural influences emanating from sources beyond the nuclear family, although the parents remain the primary interpreters and carriers of cultural attitudes about gender. These later sources of influence include teachers, athletic coaches, scout leaders, classmates, and close friends. Meyer (1982) follows a similar definition, though differing with Stoller in some respects regarding the transsexuals he (Meyer) studied clinically. Gender identity for Meyer is an earlier, more fundamental acquisition than sexual identity: "referring to a basic amalgamation of anatomical givens and reproductive potential into the self-representation" (p. 383). His concepts are derived from a massive clinical study of transsexuals and is influenced by Mahlerian theories of separation-individuation and object constancy. Coates et al. (1991), in their study of gender disorders in young boys, found that this condition "emerges in a narrow time frame and in most boys the disorder consolidates between ages 2 and 3" (p. 482). It occurs in a "context of a disturbance in the child's relational experience and experience of the self" (p. 488). The boy wishes he were a girl and dislikes being a boy. He wants to wear dresses and play with dolls. The Rorschach test reveals most commonly: "object representations were dominated by images of over controlling, overpowering, and malevolent figures" and "significant boundary disturbances" (p. 488). The mothers interfere with the son's development of autonomy and regard rough-and-tumble play as too dangerous. The father's relationship with the boy is flawed and the father is more focused on himself, requires much praise, is sensitive to narcissistic hurts; and he has temper outbursts. Most commonly the mothers were depressed by some major traumatic event such as the death of a parent or sibling, rape, serious illness, miscarriage, and threats from life-threatening illnesses. Most if not all of children with gender identity disorder (GID) become homosexual as adults if not treated.

Morrison and Severino (1997) present some rather interesting data to show that moral development proceeds along different lines in boys and girls. "Men will be concerned about measuring up to their identification with the 'masculine.' Their observing ego will use rules and principles to measure the success of their identification with father" (p. 269). The ego ideal and superego will also use rules and principles. Whereas women "will be concerned about the security of affection and maintaining affectionate relationships. Their observing ego will use affective experiences to measure the preservation of their relationship with father" (p. 269). Shame experiences, they say, are "essential for growth and differentiation to autonomy" (p. 270).

MALE GENDER IDENTITY

Tyson (1986a) has differentiated male gender development into three strands: core gender identity, gender role identity, and sexual partner orientation. She emphasized that:

> [T]he early childhood roots of gender identity, particularly as the earliest years are the time when important internal structures are established and consolidated. Later manifestations, although not the same as the early ones, have their roots in the early childhood configurations . However, the contributions to an overall broad sense of gender identity made during the latency and adolescent years must not be overlooked. The final outcome of any position along any of the strands is not finally consolidated until the end of adolescence. Indeed, adult experiences may also make important contributions [p. 423].

Friedman and Downey (1994) discuss the biological and psychoanalytic issues relative to homosexuality. Friedman (1991) states that core gender identity (CGI) takes place in most so-called normal boys and girls through "complex interactions between constitutional predisposition, and cognitive, social learning, and psychodynamic factors (i.e., identifications)" (Friedman, 1991, p. 230). Core gender identity seems well established by the age of 2 and certainly by 3 when the little boy experiences castration anxiety and early triangulation (Abelin, 1980). He is very much aware that he is male and is very proud of his body. He may even try to counterphobically reassure his mother that if she doesn't have a penis, she may grow one, or he will get one for her. Fast (1984) argues that there is an earlier, overinclusive phase of development when both sexes are not aware of sex differences or limitations inherent in their biologically and psychologically assigned gender. She says interest in the difference between the sexes begins with recognition of the limits: "the boy's interest in the mother's place in the origin of babies and the girl's recognition that she has no penis" (p. 22), and this pushes the girl to focus on feminine characteristics and being female. In general, young women tend to more readily personalize their relationships, express their subjective states directly and spontaneously, and are more self-contained, while young men are in flux and in the process of becoming (Simmel, 1984).

FEMALE GENDER IDENTITY

A revolution was created in female psychology by M. J. Sherfey's 1966 paper, "The Evolution and Nature of Female Sexuality: Relation to Psychoanalytic Theory," and it stimulated a host of responses by psychoanalysts, among whom was Benedek (1968, 1976). Outside the field, other scholars such as the physicist E. F. Keller (1982, 1983) and Harding (1987) have attacked the so-called male-dominated physical sciences as "sexist." One such claim is that girls do poorly in math classes because they feel intimidated by the boys who are more aggressive in class participation and are called on more frequently by teachers. However, when girls are segregated into classes by themselves, they do as well or better than boys. Feminists claim that women are more interested in the interrelationships of particles whereas men in science tend to focus on individual phenomena. Levin (1988), Professor of Philosophy at Yeshiva University, responded that Keller's and Harding's arguments are too harsh and epistemologically thin.

Numerous attacks on Freud and his psychoanalytic theories about female psychology from feminists and other serious critics have led to some interesting information. Thérèse Benedek's (1976) brilliant response to Strouse (1974), emphasized her psychobiological conceptual approach without making an apology for Freud's mistaken ideas. Roiphe's (1968) and Galenson and Roiphe's (1976a,b, 1979, 1980) contributions greatly increased our understanding of both male and female gender development, even though their studies follow Freud's constructions that both male and female psychological development is based on an early awareness of the penis (6 to 8 months); the awareness of sexual differences between the sexes and heightened genital awareness with masturbation and castration fears (16 to 19 months), that it is a preoedipal form of phallic exhibitionism (Edgecumbe and Burgner, 1975). Feminist scholars and feminist psychoanalysts have brought "the two fields closer and yet added to the difficulty" between the modern feminist position and the classical Freudian position (Mahfouz and Smith, 1994, p. ix).

When the little girl discovers that she doesn't possess a penis, her developing personality becomes centrally organized around this perceived fact. According to those psychoanalytic researchers who subscribe to the classical view, women develop penis envy. In some psychoanalytic circles, there is considerable doubt cast on the concept of penis envy and with the suggestion that it be dropped. However, Mayer (1995) suggests from her clinical experience of analyses of women that there must be two lines of development for female identity: one arising from the revived classical Freudian castration complex and the other from primary femininity. Specific affects are associated with these two different developmental sequences. For example, anxiety is associated with a perceived danger to the female genitalia (genital anxiety) and depression is associated with loss of the imaginary penis. Penis envy, therefore, is the clinical manifestation in numbers of competitive women who wish to be male that Mayer asserts is not incompatible with being happy as a female. She quotes Kubie (1974) to the effect that both boys and girls sometimes wish to be both sexes. She summarizes her thesis by saying that the girl has "two different tasks: coming to terms with what she *isn't* and *hasn't* even as she learns to deal with what she *is* and what she *has*" (p. 32).

Other psychoanalytic clinicians' experience, however, is that penis envy is not as universal as was formerly thought. Gender development in women, according to Tyson (1986b), arises with a constitutionally and biologically based "primary sense of being female" (p. 2) to which is added the libidinally charged oral, anal, urethral, and genital experiences of the infant–mother dyad. To this is added "cognitive maturation, especially the capacity for representational thought, the infant girl's libidinal sensations are integrated into her 'body ego' " (p. 2). This point of view is confirmed by my own observations and reconstructions of childhood from the analyses of adult women. During early infant and mother developmental experiences multiple sensory modalities (tactile, temperature, proprioceptive, auditory, olfactory, visual, etc.) contribute to the laying down of internalized complex caretaking experiences that are both optimally gratifying and mildly frustrating. Out of these experiences, an internal self representation is constructed that is uniquely female for that individual. Tyson asserts that this female self representation is formed by the age of 18 months. Cognitive development proceeds pari passu, giving rise to conscious and unconscious identificatory wishes to be " 'at one with' and 'the same as' the idealized mother" (p. 2) including having babies like mother. These wishes are revived and reinforced in the realistic setting of the married young adult woman. By this time, in the optimal case, there has been a working through of the rapprochement conflicts of ambivalence centering around separation from the mother. Tyson says, "the degree to which the adult woman can integrate genitality into her adult personality and consolidate a feminine gender identity, a feminine gender role and a feminine choice of love object, depends upon her abilities to resolve ambivalence towards her mother and selectively identify with her" (p. 10).

Tyson (1994) follows Stoller's (1985) view about gender identity and refines her rejection of the traditional view of castration anxiety and penis envy. She suggests that gender issues follow three separate "intertwining phenomena: gender identity, gender role identity, and sexual partner orientation" (p. 451). For her:

> *Gender identity*, or a sense of femininity or masculinity, refers to a broad psychological configuration that combines personal identity, biological sex, erotic sensations, interpersonal experiences , intrapsychic consequences (such as identifications) and social and cultural influences. *Gender role identity* refers to the gender-based patterning conscious and unconscious interactions with other people. *Sexual partner orientation* refers to the preferred sex of the sexual partner. Core gender identity arises by 18–24 months through an awareness of the oral, anal, urethral, and genital bodily zones leading to "a basic sense of belonging to one sex and not the other . . ." [pp. 451–452].

This core gender identity contains identifications with both parents and siblings that becomes more complex with generous and elaborate mixtures of masculine and feminine features as development proceeds through childhood and adolescence into young adulthood. Tyson contends that girls, through identification processes, have it much easier than boys because of being of the same sex as the mother. She describes some clinical material that focuses on sexual object choice issues from deeply imbedded preoedipal and oedipal conflicts with the mother and powerful angry and ambivalent relations with the mother that are accentuated by separation from her. Tyson (1994), furthermore, challenges those Freudian theorists such as Deutsch (1944), Roiphe and Galenson (1981), Galenson and Roiphe (1976b) and Mayer (1995), who have followed the classical view that when the girl discovers she doesn't possess a penis she feels castrated and envies boys. Fast (1990) is critical of classical Freudian phallocentrism as untenable. She describes three stages of development of gender development. First, from birth to 18 to 24 months is an early undifferentiated period in which the child possesses both male and female capacities, and a primary identification with both mother and father. The second stage begins at 18 to 24 months, when there is an awareness of the differences between the sexes. The third stage (differentiation proper) occurs around the oedipal period when masculine and feminine themes are expressed in the respective male and female child. Mothers and fathers aid in the differentiation process by appropriate reinforcement.

In spite of some complications arising from uncertainties regarding a girl's inner genital space (Erikson, 1964; Barnett, 1966; Kestenberg, 1968, 1980; Kirkpatrick, 1980, 1981) a strong sense of a coherent body-self is created in a girl. Barnett (1966) is even more definite about an awareness of an interior space in infancy and childhood that is primarily repressed and only later recathected through her awareness of other orifices (oral and anal) and their contents. Chodorow (1978, 1989a), like

Tyson, has argued that psychoanalytic studies of gender development in women have in the past concentrated too heavily on the male-centered concepts of the presence or absence of the penis, penis envy, or penis awe (Freud, 1931; Greenacre, 1953). "The classic Freudian account of the Oedipus complex is imbued with an inexorable logic following two basic assumptions about sex and gender: first, Freud defines gender and sexual differentiation as presence or absence of masculinity and the male genital rather than as two different presences; second, Freud maintains a functional teleological view of the 'destiny' reserved for anatomical differences between the sexes" (Chodorow, 1978, pp. 157–158). Chodorow goes on to say:

> [T]he main importance of the Oedipus complex . . . is in the constitution of different forms of relational potential in people of different genders. The Oedipus complex in the form in which the internal interpersonal world will later be imposed on and help to create the external postoedipal (and in the girl postpubertal) personality is the relatively stable foundation upon which other forms of relational development will build [1978, p. 166].

She also emphasizes the effects that the infant has on the mother, which echoes Benedek's concept of parenthood as a developmental phase (1959, 1970). Chodorow, however, has arrived at this notion from a social science perspective that, while it is very instructive, lacks the affirming clinical resonance that Benedek's work brings. Furthermore, Chodorow's object relations theoretical perspective eliminates other points of view that may be useful and explanatory. Chodorow emphasizes the fact that the dyadic relationship between mother and daughter continues, with cycles of separation and merger, on into young adulthood. There is a primary identification with the mother and a fusion of identification and object choice, whereas boys are pushed out of this intimate preoedipal relationship with the mother. Girls, on the other hand, emerge from this with a stronger sense of empathy in experiencing the feelings of others, but are less differentiated than boys. In effect, girls do not "resolve" their Oedipus complex like boys do, and remain attached to their mothers while retaining an oedipal attachment to father. Chodorow (1989b) also is influenced by psychoanalytic feminism (Sayers, 1986). Chodorow focuses on "an open web of social, psychological, and cultural relations, dynamics, practices, identities, beliefs, in which I would privilege neither society, psyche, nor culture [that] comes to constitute gender as a social, cultural, and psychological phenomenon" (1989b, p. 5). However, since she has gotten into psychoanalytic training, she has been drawn to object relations theory to explain her sociologically informed observations.

In her discussion of Chodorow's paper (1989a), Rocah (1989) also advocated a pluralistic approach to the study of gender to include both psychodynamic and sociological issues, forming a kind of gestalt. But Rocah, like Freud (1925), would emphasize the child's early awareness of the anatomical differences between the sexes. (As noted above, one 3-year-old boy said to his mother that he "knew she didn't have a penis, but not to worry, he would get her one.") Hurn (1969) described the complex processes of identification of the male child with the father and how fatherhood enhances the man's development, while Rocah (1984) has described the mutual influences of mother and daughter. Galatzer-Levy's (1984) rich clinical data about the dyadic processes in the breakdown of either parent or adolescent and the effects on each other, are important contributions to this area of research. Even earlier, M. Balint (1949) and later Mahler (1969; Mahler, Pine, and Bergman, 1975) borrowed from biology the term *symbiosis* to describe these same processes between mother and child. However, psychoanalytic contributions in this area have been all too few. The role of the father with his children (Ross, 1975, 1983) has been elaborated, along with the development of his own paternal identity. Brody and Axelrod (1978), Lamb (1976), and Cath, Gurwitt, and Gunsberg (1989) have also made significant contributions to this area. Abelin's (1975, 1980) construction of "early triangulation" is another widely accepted formulation of the developmental sequences occurring in the practicing subphase of separation-individuation (18 months). The father's role in "specific refueling" with the infant is very important in this development. Later on in latency and adolescence, the father's action-oriented activities are very important in identification processes in the male, while his acceptance and mirroring of the daughter's budding sexuality facilitates the development of her sexual and gender identity (see also Weissman [1963] and an attractive book of photographs of fathers with their children [Reich, 1960]). Slipp (1993) speculates about Freud's early development to explain his faulty understanding of female gender development. Losses during Freud's early separation–individuation period of his Nanny, the emotional loss of his mother, and the death of his brother Julius, led to his ambivalent attitudes toward women. If one follows this point of view, the often quoted reason that Freud was greatly influenced by the Viennese fin de siecle culture is thus somewhat diminished.

The development of identity patterns of college people and especially women (Josselman, 1980, 1989; see chapter 2) shows that separation–individuation issues are most important in determining the outcome of the developmental tasks of young adults. In fact, the most salient conclusion from Josselson's study is that identity development in women is critically determined by the relative degree of resolution of a young woman's conflicts about separating from her parents, especially her mother, during late adolescence, and more so in young adulthood. From a clinical psychoanalytic perspective, Tyson (1982,

1986a,b,c, 1989, 1994), Galenson and Roiphe (1976a,b, 1979, 1980), and from a theoretical and sociological perspective, Chodorow (1978, 1989a,b) have arrived at the same conclusions. One young adult woman regularly relived her developmental conflicts with her mother in her relationships with her male employers whom she perceived to be dominating and with an irrational insistence on always being right.

Another all too common case in point is when some young women struggle to separate themselves from their mothers (and fathers), following graduation from college or involvement in other groups. In fact, there has been a trend for a number of years now of young people moving back with their parents for economic reasons, especially in large metropolitan areas like New York City, Los Angeles, and Chicago where rents are high. So, whilst it may not be an ideal situation, it is surely common enough throughout the country and across socioeconomic classes. For these women serious difficulty in finding a suitable vocation to support themselves has led to severe shame and humiliation in failing in this developmental task. The parents usually intervene when this emergency situation requires that the young person move back into the family home. Predictably, the move promotes the regressive reactivation of earlier adolescent issues. Partially resolved conflicts of rapprochement and separation–individuation issues reappear, which is disruptive and painful for all concerned. Affective storms of anxiety, rage, and reciprocally experienced guilt are frequent occurrences.

Psychoanalytic therapy is indicated, and is usually quite helpful, but in some less pathological instances what can make a critical difference is the felicitous experience of an appropriate choice of a love object that in the case of heterosexuals eventually leads to marriage. In the best of circumstances, what such examples demonstrate is that late adolescent and young adulthood development is often incomplete until the reality of reexperiencing a new loving relationship with a potential mate adds the missing ingredient. A suitable and satisfying "this-is-me" kind of vocation can produce a more solid personality consolidation, too. Notable also is the insight that sometimes a stable sexual relationship contributes significantly to the overall development of a cohesive personality in late adolescence and young adulthood, specifically to identity formation. But for some individuals, though, it is not clear that a satisfying sexual relationship is absolutely essential for stable personality development. What is clear from clinical experience is that conflicts about sexual feelings and sexual behavior definitely can and often do interfere with a solid consolidation of the personality and identity formation. What is explicit here in this chapter is the relevance of intimacy in terms of sexual behavior patterns to identity formation and identity cohesion. Men sometimes separate from the nuclear family with less conflict and ambivalence, but overall, women tend to have more conflicts about separating from parents.

Sexual identity is reflected in sexual behavior patterns or sexual orientation. In adolescence and young adulthood, experimental efforts in establishing and consolidating sexual and gender identities, which began much earlier in childhood, are reflected (Tyson, 1982, 1986a,b, 1989, 1994; Fast, 1984, 1990). The sexual patterns, which settle out from various experiments in object (re)finding (Freud, 1905, p. 222, 1909, 1915, 1917, 1924), and object ongoing relationships during adolescence, may not be the final patterns of sexual behavior in late adolescence and young adulthood. These patterns resemble those that Laufer (1976) and Ritvo (Panel, 1987, p. 184) referred to as centrally organizing sexual fantasies. In my own clinical experience, these same type of fantasies as reconstructed from the analyses of adults, make their first appearance in either oedipal, latency, or pubertal age children, but then crystallize into more enduring, structuralized, and repeatable patterns of sexual behavior during middle adolescence, late adolescence, and young adulthood. This observation seems to be true for both heterosexual and homosexual styles of behavior. For example, one adult man's unconscious sexual fantasies from early to middle adolescence, centered around a cute girl small enough for him to physically pick up. Another man's recovered and constructed unconscious masturbation fantasy involved tying up a sexually starved woman so that she was helplessly submissive and begging to be sexually overwhelmed by him. A third example is of a man whose frustrated sexual tensions were relieved by looking at nude women dancers that reminded him of his nude mother parading around the house. Sexual identity, however, must be differentiated from *gender identity*, a term that refers to those unique combinations of masculine and feminine qualities and characteristics present in any individual. The term *sexual identity* refers to biological and physiological maleness and femaleness.

SEXUAL IDENTITY

Sexual identity receives a major boost during the oedipal and adolescent phases of development and is "marked by the acquisition of the qualities of masculinity, femininity, and eroticism which are expressed in sexual fantasies, attractions, and object choices. Sexual identity at any given developmental level is ordinarily a refinement of basic gender sense in terms of personal eroticism and conventional as well as idiosyncratic expressions of masculinity and femininity" (Meyer, 1982, p. 383). Sexual identity is a complex structure since it is determined by a multitude of physical and biological factors. To obtain a thorough evaluation of sexual identity (following Stoller's suggestion), one must assay the sex chromosomes, concentrations of sex hormones in the body fluids, examine the internal sexual organs (uterus, prostate, gonads, etc.), external genitalia, as well as the secondary sex characteristics. These physiological and biological influences obviously have psychological meanings which are important at each phase of development, but sexual orientation (heterosexual or homosexual) has very complex origins and psychoanalytic investigation of unconscious fantasy life is an important contribution. Moreover, sexual object choice does not simply rest on Freud's famous triad of source, aim, and object. Social, cultural, and biological influences can play important influences as well. Moreover, it is clear that careful study of the patterns of sexual behavior in longitudinal and in-depth biopsychosocial research of both sexes is necessary before specific explanatory expositions can be made about sexual identity.

Recent molecular biological studies (Haqq, King, Ukiyama, Falsafi, Haqq, Donahoe, and Weiss, 1994) have shown that the SRY gene on the short arm of the Y chromosome, stimulates the production of testosterone by the Leydig cells that in turn activate the Mullerian Inhibiting Substance (MIS), secreted by the Sertoli cells, to produce regression of the Mullerian Duct that is the anlagen of the uterus, Fallopian tubes, and upper vagina. These embryological events take place at around 35 weeks of gestation producing a male, but if not, then the primary female fetus continues to develop. Mutations in this complex process lead to sex reversal, male hermaphroditism, and retained Mullerian duct syndrome. In an earlier study of mammalian brain embryogenesis, MacLusky and Naftolin (1981) showed that testosterone is converted into estrogens to masculinize the brain, while in the female brain estrogens are possibly blocked by a plasma estrogen-binding system or progesterone.

HOMOSEXUAL IDENTITY (OR ORIENTATION) PATTERNS

Friedman (1988) has introduced a refreshingly new approach, including a biopsychosocial approach, that takes into account

much of the biological and neuroscience research that has revolutionized the study of sexual orientation in recent years
(Friedman and Downey, 1993, 1994). He defines sexual orientation as a very complex set of factors that include one's subjective sense of being heterosexual, homosexual, or bisexual.
Prenatal and postnatal hormonal levels and social psychological issues influence the outcome of a whole range of behaviors
in boys' discomfort in body image as being unmasculine or in
girls as being too masculine. In a sociological study, Deisher
(1989) found that 10 percent of the estimated 30 million people in the 10 to 20 age group consider themselves exclusively
or predominately homosexual. But this figure has been dis-
puted by the monumental study at the University of Chicago
(Michael, Gagnon, Laumann, and Kolata, 1994): Their figures
are 3 to 5 percent. Whatever the actual percentages, Troiden's
study (1989) of this age group revealed a four-stage process:
sensitization, identity confusion, identity assumption, and
commitment. This model takes into account finding and identifying with an existing group that solidifies an evolving self-
definition. In the *sensitization* stage during childhood and preadolescence, potential homosexuals feel different and are puzzled by that experience. There is not much joy in same-sex
activities such as rough and tumble sports in males and playing
with dolls, jumping rope, playing house, and hopscotch in females, leading to the experience of feeling out of step with
their peers (Herdt, 1989). The significance of the sensitization
experiences rests in the meanings attached to these feelings
later on in adolescence when sexual maturation evolves. The
second stage, *identity confusion,* follows when childhood experiences are endowed in middle and late adolescence with sexual
meaning along with sexual arousal experiences, much misin-
formation about homosexuality, and the stigma associated with
it. In fact, homosexual late adolescents learn to "hide"
through an elaborate set of defenses such as dating women who

accept for whatever reason a platonic, nonsexual, or friendship relationship (Martin, 1982). Lesbians reach this stage later than males by a few years. The third stage, *identity assumption,* occurs in gay males on the average at age 19 to 21; females, at 21 to 23. With men, assumption of a homosexual identity occurs in the context of sexual encounters with other men, while with women it occurs more in the context of an emotional relationship with another woman. The fourth stage, *commitment,* involves engaging in a love relationship with more "self-acceptance and comfort with the homosexual identity and role" (p. 63).

Margaret Schneider (1989) studied the sexual identities of some individuals in the Toronto lesbian community. She classified five categories: growing awareness of homosexual feelings and identity; positive evaluation of homosexuality; developing intimate same-sex romantic/erotic relationships; establishing social ties with gay peers; and self-disclosure. These stages parallel the adolescent process and are interrelated. Adolescent lesbians usually avoid socializing tasks rather than proceeding with them. Additionally, it is very difficult for younger mid-adolescent 15-year-old lesbians to declare themselves because they feel out of place with older 25-year-old young adult lesbians in an adult environment. Legal age of consent issues are also involved in relationships between 15-year-olds and those ten years older.

As cogent as the above observations are, Boxer and Cohler (1989) raise some seriously provocative questions and advise caution in interpreting the data from subjects' recall of memories of childhood and adolescence in an informal nonclinical setting. Narrative life course studies (Offer and Offer, 1975; Levinson, Darrow, Klein, Levinson, and McKee, 1978) have been especially near-sighted in dealing with the complexities of the lives of nonclinical cohorts. As valuable as these studies can be in a sociopsychological sense, Boxer and Cohler (1989):

[A]rgue for the necessity for prospective, longitudinal, life-span investigations (employing both predictive and interpretive methodologies), which will have an impact not only on our understanding of vulnerability, resilience, and well-being of gay and lesbian youth as well as for adults, but also carry important implications for models, methods and theories within the social sciences for the study of [gay] lives" [p. 320].

The questions Boxer and Cohler (1989) raise are: What is the effect of the AIDS crisis on adjustment to the transition into adulthood? What kind of socialization processes result from the help offered to a few gay and lesbian adolescents by various social services agencies? Qualitative and quantitative studies are necessary to tease out the many variables that are special for gay and lesbian youth, since they are also negotiating the developmental tasks all adolescents and young adults are confronted with. The reciprocal effects of offspring on parents over time have not been sufficiently studied either (Cook and Cohler, 1986). "It remains an open question as to what subsequently happens to those who are physically or emotionally abused by friends, family, or society at large" (p. 341). But gay and lesbian adolescents would certainly appear to be at high risk for drug abuse, prostitution, sexually transmitted diseases, and various psychosocial disorders including manifestly psychiatric illnesses because of prior traumatic experiences.

Isay (1986), from his clinical psychoanalytic observations, derives three broad stages of development of homosexual identity formation in men: "a childhood acquisition stage, the consolidation stage of adolescence and early adulthood, and the integration stage of adulthood" (p. 487).

LITERARY CONTRIBUTIONS

Literary characters offer some special insights into issues of sexual identity. For example, the pure, sweet virginal innocence of Margarete in the opera *Faust* (Barbier and Carre,

1859) is contrasted with the earthy, seductive, and rebellious central character in the opera *Carmen* (Meilhac and Halevy, 1875). The sexual behavior of the two women resembles two clinically observed patterns that evolve in adolescence and become consolidated in late adolescence and young adulthood. Dr. Faustus sold his soul in order to regain and revel in a narcissistically idealized youthful sexual freedom without any regard for Margarete's commitment to the ideals of virginity and marital love that eventually led to her losing her life. Such narcissistic and self-serving behavior became a dominant theme of the sexual revolution in the adolescent and young adult populations in the United States in the 1960s, 1970s, and 1980s. In the 1990s the scare of AIDS has slowed that revolution considerably in both heterosexual and homosexual populations, although the fastest growing population afflicted with immune deficiency diseases includes women and children.

On the other hand, the character of Carmen is not at all fearful of publicly proclaiming her philosophy of free love. In so doing, she seduces Don Jose away from his mother's chaste female messenger, Micsela. Moreover, Carmen's saucy behavior of giving Don Jose a flower is understood to be symbolic of her freedom to be sexual.

In the same vein, the legendary exploits and the problems generated by the patterns of Don Juan's mythic (Pratt, 1960) sexual behavior have been immortalized in Tirso de Molina's (1630) classic version of the play *Don Juan* and in Spanish *El Burlador de Sevilla (The Mocker of Seville*; see also chapter 5). Paul Monette (1992) has written a sensitive, poignant, and clinically authentic life story (probably autobiographical) of a very troubled person who struggled to overcome a serious gender and sexual identity disorder. His sexual conflicts were all entangled with guilt about his homosexual feelings from early childhood, and further complicated by shame about his failed efforts to convert to a heterosexual lifestyle. He was exquisitely afraid of the dangers of intimacy with both men and women. At the end of the book, he had apparently found love and affection with a man of similar interests and with whom he was for the most part compatible. His story resonates with that of so many gay people and emphasizes the fact that many gay men must struggle to achieve a solid sense of selfhood.

Dalsimer's (1986) interpretation of Jane Austen's novel, *Persuasion* (1818), demonstrates how thoroughly Austen understood the issues of parent loss. Dalsimer points out how the character Anne dealt with loss of her mother first in early adolescence and was persuaded to turn down an offer of marriage in late adolescence at age 19. In the end, it was a resolution of the mourning surrounding these losses that allowed her to move on into adulthood, reject her surrogate mother's advice, leave her family, and finally accept the marriage offer she had refused earlier.

Cahill's (1988) study of women writers writing about their mothers offers a special insight into their relationship. For example, Virginia Woolf's mother died at age 49 when Virginia was 13. At 44, she wrote *To the Lighthouse* (1927) in a rush and afterwards was no longer so obsessed with her mother's death and her mother's "quick temper" and the fact that she was "hardly an image of warmth and empathy" (Wolf and Wolf, 1979, p. 42). She wrote: "I suppose I did for myself what psychoanalysts do for their patients. I expressed in some way long felt and deeply felt emotions. And in expressing it I explained it and then laid it to rest" (p. 313). She asked herself if, by explaining her feelings, her "vision" and "feeling" for her mother became dimmer, but still in this "Sketch of the Past" from "Moments of Being" compared painting a portrait of her mother's personality as being as hard as painting a Cezanne (p. 319). Virginia Woolf measured her mother's character in terms of the two men she married: "one, the pink of propriety; the other, the pink of intellectuality" (p. 320). The memories of kissing her mother's still warm face and later kissing the cold face, along with the intense smell of flowers, remained powerful well into adulthood. Yet another literary study by Gilbert and Gubar (1979) of Emily Dickinson's literary development includes her grasp of a gender and sexual identity that is both gothic and romantic, particularly her "self-hauntings of (female) gothic fiction are in Dickinson's view essential to (female) art" (pp. 585–586).

SOCIOLOGICAL ISSUES

A special issue of the *Journal of Youth and Adolescence* (June 1987) was devoted to the study of sex and gender issues in regard to family (psychosocial) relations during adolescence. Current studies indicating that there are no significant or consistent differences in the family relations of boys and girls (Hauser, Book, Houlihan, Powers, Weiss-Perry, Follansbee, Jacobson, and Noam, 1987) suggests that the "case for sex differences has been overstated" (Steinberg, 1987, p. 194). However, identity development does differ in boys and girls, as Steinberg quotes Bronfenbrenner's (1961) findings that "healthy psychosocial development among young women may require more of a concerted effort to establish autonomy in family relations; among young men, however, the same goal may require maintaining more connectedness in the family" (Steinberg, 1987, pp. 194–195). More importantly, it seems there are major differences between parenting behavior of mothers and fathers vis-à-vis their children. "For example, Hauser et al. found that fathers are more likely to be cognitively enabling and involved in problem solving in family discussions, while mothers are more likely to interrupt, to distract, and to interfere. Perhaps as a consequence, the authors speculate, adolescents—males and females alike—are more likely to direct their discourse toward fathers than toward mothers" (Steinberg, 1987, p. 195).

On the other hand, McDermott, Waldron, Char, Ching, Izatsu, Mann, Ponce, and Fukuanga (1987) found that young adult men and women continue to regard their mothers as the major support figure of the family, which is a continuation of what they felt in adolescence. The father is regarded by sons as the source of power in both phases of development, while women do not differentiate between mothers and fathers in terms of power roles. According to the authors, one possible implication of this study is that women appear to be separating from their families more rapidly than men. Another interpretation is that since women now enjoy more opportunities for professional and business careers, they feel freer to seek out their fathers as sources for identification with his power and masculine aggressiveness, since such qualities are very useful in advancing themselves in their careers. However, I am not referring here to the sad fact that 55 percent of employed women still work in service type jobs, in the so-called "pink ghetto."

In general, young adult women tend to more readily personalize their relationships, express their subjective states directly and spontaneously, and are more self-contained, while young men are in flux and transition of becoming (Simmel, 1984). In my own experience, the father is more involved where money and power issues are concerned, while dating problems and setting limits about heterosexual relations are negotiated between daughters and mothers.

CLINICAL DATA

During latency, one man drew pictures of nude women to stimulate and at the same time soothe himself, and later on in young adulthood he sought out prostitutes and frequented stripper joints to relieve tensions that were derived from a deep longing for contact with his mother who was cold, withdrawn, and depressed. The analysis revealed that he was attempting to restore the only situation he knew of closeness with his mother—viewing her nude body that she frequently exposed to him. Both parents were cold, unloving people who withheld support and encouragement from their children, while the father loudly touted his own accomplishments. Photographs of the mother from this period of his childhood reveal a depressed, tense, and withdrawn woman.

During preadolescence and later in adolescence, a boy admiringly pored over pictures of muscular men while stimulating himself, but when his "secret" was discovered he was put to shame with depreciatingly experienced comments that called his gender into question. Later on in young adulthood, he sought out persons who represented for him the ideal body build, but more importantly what was added were new interests in emotional, intellectual, and cultural values.

A young adult man was very proud of his lean prizefighter-like muscular physique that he enjoyed exhibiting to other men at the health club. He was motivated to engage in a strenuous training program to counteract a shame-induced, conscious memory of his slight body image during latency and adolescence. That his adult muscular physical appearance be noticed and admired was important to maintaining a cohesive self-regard. Phallic narcissistic and exhibitionistic meanings were not repressed but conflicted with persistent earlier self representations. He was equally proud of his professional and creatively artistic accomplishments.

The sexual pattern begun in a young woman's middle phase of adolescence consisted of a marked inhibition and identification with the perceived values of her mother that healthy sex was the lesser of life's goals. Fear of the mother's criticism, and adoption of her mother's identity as an underprivileged woman, interfered with a full appreciation of her sexuality and the realization of her potentialities. She was left with an unresolved, rivalrous oedipal conflict that underwent significant resolution in the analysis of her fears and guilt feelings surfacing around separation from her mother. Breaking with her mother's rigid and severe views about sexuality was relived in the transference neurosis.

Mark was the only boy in an Italian family, which automatically made him the family favorite. He was so cute and cuddly all the women in the family wanted to have him sit on their laps. The mother clung to him in her depressed state, and his grandmother and aunts were only slightly outdone by her. Such overstimulation set him apart in childhood and latency, but puberty, appearing as early as it did at 10 or 11, gave powerful hormonal and overwhelming physiological impetus to his developing sexuality. One outlet was early masturbation and exhibiting himself to the girl next door. The parents tried to curb this behavior by warning him that he would turn out like one of the lurid sexual murderers then prominently displayed in the newspapers. But when he had nocturnal erections and emissions, it was very difficult to hide these developments from his parents. As a teenager he was timid with girls, until he met his wife to be, with whom he has been sexually active ever since late adolescence. What brought him to analysis were repeated bouts of depression and a pervasive sense of guilt that set the stage for the formation of his identity.

Passivity was a major defense against his guilt feelings which were constantly being replenished by a vivid fantasy life. Feelings of helplessness, and the ensuing depressions, completed the clinical picture. His identity as a sexually depraved or perverted person persisted well into adulthood, since he experienced his lively sexual fantasies as very dominating and overwhelming themes early on in the analysis. He was tempted to act on these fantasies, but they seemed at first to serve a defensive function. When this was interpreted, he felt less pressure to act on them. To be sure, this case did not involve a disorder of the inner self. Rather, his sexual fantasies bolstered his lowered self-esteem associated with his depression and feelings of helplessness. Competitive rivalry with his father as repeated in the transference constituted the essence of his unconscious conflicts about success, in spite of much professional and business success.

Sarah lost both parents in an automobile accident at the age of 14. Like a young adolescent, she was inhibited sexually. This was graphically demonstrated in a dream in which she wore a yellow knit bikini, but in the second part of the dream young children were attacked by a mob with shards of glass, piercing their bodies. Her associations led us to conclude that she was wishing to be freer sexually but she was very afraid of availing herself of a meaningful sexual relationship. The connection of the dangers of sexual freedom with the automobile accident is patently clear from the second part of the dream where children's bodies were pierced by shards of glass. Her interests in sexual freedom produced such anxiety and guilt that she was in constant conflict and her whole emotional life suffered. Having fun was equated with being free of her parents' control. But even more importantly, it meant the death of her parents. There was no one there to help her deal with her adolescent concerns about sexuality. At age 16, her older sister with whom she lived, refused to iron her prom dress, claiming she had to be more independent and be more self-sufficient. What made this incident all the more poignant and painfully recalled was that she was to be especially honored at the school dance as the designated Queen.

As a young adult she converted all relationships with men, including the transference with her analyst, into simulated mother relationships. Throughout adolescence she didn't have a mother or a surrogate for that matter. Her older sister could have served in this capacity, but unfortunately she suffered the additional tragedy of losing her husband in yet another automobile accident. The sister was a poor substitute for mother since she was grieving for both parents and husband. As the sister gradually emerged from mourning her losses, she was partially able to respond to Sarah's need for appropriate mirroring. But Sarah's identity was, in part, that of an abandoned, unwanted, angry, and alienated person. She was incredulously surprised and shocked that men found her attractive since she wore casual bulky clothing that obscured her feminine figure. At the same time, she had never been without a steady boyfriend since adolescence. Another part of her identity included a grandiose notion that she was rich and entitled to the life of international travel and high living without any concerns for money. As the angry, ambivalent mother transference was worked through, she was able to begin to mourn the loss of her parents and begin to relate more realistically and effectively with men. She secured a job more in keeping with her personality skills and intellect. She remembered, too, that she had been her father's favorite.

One young adult woman saw herself as the ugly duckling who could not compete successfully with her strikingly beautiful mother. This perception was made all the more poignant when her boyfriends were greeted at the door by the full-bosomed mother in her low-cut blouse. Even though she had a successful marriage to a very desirable professional man, she was still involved in a very competitive and rivalrous relationship with her mother. She persistently felt ugly and unattractive as compared to her mother. Much analytic work with her unconscious rage with the mother, a rage that rebounded in the form of a punitive anxiety and serious difficulties in finishing her graduate degree, led to a greater understanding of the oedipal nature of her difficulties. Moreover, as she succeeded in working through the mother transference, she discovered she could be assertive and feminine in her own way. Her intellectual skills blossomed. She became pregnant and took on the familiar glow of pregnancy. Then she was able to finish her degree, give birth to her first child, and successfully terminate her analysis all at the same time.

SUMMARY

Definitions of sexual identity, gender identity, and sexual orientation have clarified the complexity involved in the multifactorial psychological, developmental, physiological, and sociological issues of these important distinctions. Psychosexual differentiation begins in the prenatal period of embryonic development in a complex interaction of hormones, chromosomes, genes, and environmental influences (Money and Ehrhardt, 1972). Sexual orientation can be heterosexual or homosexual and is not necessarily pathological unless psychological maladaptations are observed. Gender identity disorders include perversions, transsexuality, and fetishistic behavior. Disorders in any of these conditions must be evaluated from biological, sociological, and psychological perspectives.

There has been much controversy about female sexual and gender identity beginning with Freud's early attempts, but modern research has shed considerable light on this challenging area of female development, particularly the work of women psychoanalysts. Separation issues are very important in the development of identity patterns in young adults, and critically so in young women by the relative degree of resolution of ambivalence toward parents and especially toward their mothers. The sexual identity in lesbians may be classified as a growing awareness of homosexual feelings, positive evaluation of homosexuality, developing intimate same-sex romantic–erotic relationships, establishing social ties with gay peers, and self-disclosure (Schneider, 1989).

As much as is known about both male and female homosexuality, more research must be done to establish a more solid foundation of understanding of the various homosexualities. Prospective, longitudinal, life-span studies will help us to evualate vulnerabilities, resilience, and the well-being of gay and lesbian young adults (Boxer and Cohler, 1989).

Literary, sociological, and clinical observations add significant substance to the theoretical and biological material presented in this chapter, as well as the role of the father in gender and sexual identity development (Cath et al., 1989).

REFERENCES

Abelin, E. L. (1975), Some further observations and comments on the earliest role of the father. *Internat. J. Psycho-Anal.,* 56:293–232.

———— (1980), Triangulation, the role of the father and the origins of core identity during the rapprochement subphase. In: *Rapprochement: The Critical Subphase of Separation-Individuation,* ed. R. F. Lax, S. Bach, & J. A. Burland. New York: Jason Aronson, pp. 151–169.

Austen, J. (1818), *Persuasion.* New York: Penguin, 1978.

Balint, M. (1949), Early developmental states of the ego: Primary object love. *Internat. J. Psycho-Anal.,* 30:265–273.

Barbier, J., & Carre, M. (1859), *Faust,* Libretto for Charles Guonod's Opera, tr. G. Mead. New York: G. Schirmer.

Barnett, M. (1966), Vaginal awareness in infancy and childhood of girls. *J. Amer. Psychoanal. Assn.,* 14:129–141.

Benedek, T. (1959), Parenthood as a developmental phase. *J. Amer. Psychoanal. Assn.,* 7:389–417.

———— (1968), Discussion of Sherfey's paper on female sexuality. *J. Amer. Psychoanal. Assn.,* 16:424–448.

———— (1970), Parenthood during the life cycle. In: *Parenthood: Its Psychology and Psychopathology,* ed. E. J. Anthony & T. Benedek. Boston: Little, Brown, pp. 185–206.

———— (1976), On the psychobiology of gender identity. *Annual of Psychoanalysis,* 4:117–162. New York: International Universities Press.

Bettelheim, B. (1954), *Symbolic Wounds: Puberty Rites and the Envious Male.* New York: Free Press.

Boxer, A. M., & Cohler, B. (1989), The life course of gay and lesbian youth: An immodest proposal for the study of lives. In: *Gay and Lesbian Youth,* ed. G. Herdt. Binghamton, NY: Harrington Park Press, pp. 315–355.

Brody, S., & Axelrod, S. (1978), *Mothers, Fathers, and Children.* New York: International Universities Press.

Bronfenbrenner, A. (1961), Some familial antecedents of responsibility and leadership in adolescents. In: *Leadership and Interpersonal Behavior,* ed. L. Petrullo & B. Bass. New York: Holt, Reinhart & Winston, pp. 239–271.

Cahill, S., Ed. (1988), *Mothers: Memories, Dreams, and Reflections by Literary Daughters.* New York: New American Library/Dutton.

Cath, S. H., Gurwitt, A., & Gunsberg, L. (1989), *Fathers and Their Families.* Hillside, NJ: Analytic Press.

Chodorow, N. (1978), *The Reproduction of Mothering.* Berkeley: University of California Press.

—— (1989a), What is the relation between the psychoanalytic psychology of women and psychoanalytic feminism. *The Annual of Psychoanalysis,* 17:215–242. Hillsdale, NJ: Analytic Press.

—— (1989b), *Feminism and Psychoanalytic Theory.* New Haven, CT: Yale University Press.

Coates, S., Friedman, R. C., & Wolf, S. (1991), Etiology of boyhood gender identity disorder: A model for integrating temperament, development, and psychodynamics. *Psychoanal. Dial.,* 1:481–523.

Cook, J. A., & Cohler, B. J. (1986), Reciprocal socialization and the care of offspring with cancer and with schizophrenia. In: *Life-Span Developmental Psychology: Intergenerational Relations,* ed. N. Datan, A. L. Greene, & H. W. Reese. Hillsdale, NJ: Erlbaum, pp. 223–243.

Dalsimer, K. (1986), *Female Adolescence: Psychoanalytic Reflections on Literature.* New Haven, CT: Yale University Press.

Deisher, R. W. (1989), Adolescent homosexuality: Preface. In: *Gay and Lesbian Youth,* ed. G. Herdt. Binghamton, NY: Harrington Park Press, pp. xiii-xv.

Deutsch, H. (1944), *The Psychology of Women: A Psychoanalytic Interpretation,* Vol. 1. New York: Grune & Stratton.

Diamond, M., & Sigmundson, K. (1997), Sex reassignment at birth. *Arch. Pediatr. Adolesc. Med.,* 151:298–304.

Edgecumbe, R., & Burgner, M. (1975), The phallic narcissistic phase: A differentiation between preoedipal and oedipal aspects of phallic development. *The Psychoanalytic Study of the Child,* 30:161–180. New Haven, CT: Yale University Press.

Erikson, E. (1964), Womanhood and inner space. In: *The Woman in America,* ed. R. J. Lifton. Boston: Houghton Mifflin, pp. 1–26.

Fast, I. (1984), *Gender Identity, a Differentiation Model Advances in Psychoanalysis: Theory, Research, and Practice,* Vol. 2. Hillsdale, NJ: Analytic Press.

—— (1990), Aspects of early gender development: Toward a reformulation. *Psychoanal. Psychology.* 7 (Suppl.):105–117.

Freud, S. (1905), Three Essays on the Theory of Sexuality. *Standard Edition,* 7:123–243. London: Hogarth Press, 1953.

——— (1909), Analysis of a phobia in a five-year-old boy. *Standard Edition*, 10:1–147. London: Hogarth Press, 1955.

——— (1915), Instincts and their vicissitudes. *Standard Edition*, 14:109–140. London: Hogarth Press, 1957.

——— (1917), Mourning and melancholia. *Standard Edition*, 14:237–258. London: Hogarth Press, 1957.

——— (1918), From the history of an infantile neurosis. *Standard Edition*, 17:1–122. London: Hogarth Press, 1955.

——— (1923), The Ego and the Id. *Standard Edition*, 19:1–59. London: Hogarth Press, 1961.

——— (1924), The dissolution of the Oedipus complex. *Standard Edition*, 19:171–179. London: Hogarth Press, 1961.

——— (1925), Some psychical consequences of the anatomical differences between the sexes. *Standard Edition*, 19:241–258. London: Hogarth Press, 1961.

——— (1931), Female sexuality. *Standard Edition*, 21:221–243. London: Hogarth Press, 1961.

Friedman, R. C. (1988), *Male Homosexuality*. New Haven, CT: Yale University Press.

——— (1991), *Male Homosexuality: A Contemporary Psychoanalytic Perspective*. New Haven, CT: Yale University Press.

——— Downey, J. (1993), Psychoanalysis, psychobiology, and homosexuality. *J. Amer. Psychoanal. Assn.*, 41:1159–1198.

——— ——— (1994), Homosexuality. *New Eng. J. Med.*, 331:923–930.

Galatzer-Levy, R. M. (1984), Adolescent breakdown and middle age crises. In: *Late Adolescence: Psychoanalytic Studies*, ed. D. D. Brockman. New York: International Universities Press, pp. 29–51.

Galenson, E., & Roiphe, H. (1976a), The impact of sexual discovery on mood, defensive organization and symbolization. *The Psychoanalytic Study of the Child*, 26:195–216. Chicago: Quadrangle.

——— (1976b), Some suggested revisions concerning early female development. *J. Amer. Psychoanal. Assn.*, 24 (Suppl.):29–57.

——— ——— (1979), Development of sexual identity: Discoveries and implications. In: *On Sexuality*, ed. T. B. Karasu & C. W. Socarides. New York: International Universities Press, pp. 1–17.

——— ——— (1980), The preoedipal development of the boy. *J. Amer. Psychoanal. Assn.*, 28:805–829.

Gilbert, S. M., & Gubar, S. (1979), A woman-white: "Emily Dickinson's yarn of pearl." In: *The Mad Woman in the Attic*. New Haven, CT: Yale University Press.

Greenacre, P. (1953), Penis awe and its relation to penis envy, In: *Drives, Affects, Behavior*, ed. R. M. Loewenstein. New York: International Universities Press, pp. 176–190.

Greenson, R. R. (1964), On homosexuality and gender identity. *Internat. J. Psycho-Anal.*, 45:217–219.

——— (1966), A transvestite boy and a hypothesis. *Internat. J. Psycho-Anal.*, 47:396–403.

——— (1968), Disidentifying from mother: Its special importance for the boy. *Internat. J. Psycho-Anal.*, 49:370–374.

Haber, C. H. (1991), The psychoanalytic treatment of a preschool boy with a gender identity disorder. *J. Amer. Psychoanal. Assn.*, 39:107–130.

Haqq, C. M., King, C., Ukiyama, E., Falsafi, S., Haqq, T. N., Donahoe, P. K., & Weiss, M. A. (1994), Molecular basis of mammalian sexual determination: Activation of Mullerian inhibiting substance gene expression by SRY. *Science*, 266:1494–1500.

Harding, S. (1987), The instability of the analytical categories of feminist theory. The curious coincidence of feminine and African moralities. In: *Women and Moral Theory*, ed. E. Kittay & D. Meyers. Totowa, NJ: Rowman & Littlefield, pp. 296–315.

Hauser, S. T., Book, B. K., Houlihan, J., Powers, S., Weiss-Perry, B., Follansbee, D., Jacobson, A. M., & Noam, G. (1987). Sex differences within the family: Studies of adolescent and parent family interactions. *J. Youth & Adol.*, 16:199–220.

Herdt, G. (1989), Introduction: Gay and lesbian youth, emergent identities, and cultural scenes at home and abroad. In: *Gay and Lesbian Youth*, ed. G. Herdt. Binghampton, NY: Harrington Park Press, pp. 1–42.

Hurn, H. (1969), Synergic relations between the processes of fatherhood and psychoanalysis. *J. Amer. Psychoanal. Assn.*, 17:437–451.

Isay, R. A. (1986), The development of sexual identity in homosexual men. *The Psychoanalytic Study of the Child*, 41:467–489. New Haven, CT: Yale University Press.

Josselson, R. (1980), Ego development in adolescence. In: *Handbook of Adolescent Psychology*, ed. J. Adelson. New York: John Wiley, pp. 188–210.

——— (1989), Identity formation in adolescence: Implications for young adulthood. In: *Adolescent Psychiatry*, 16:142–154. Chicago: University of Chicago Press.

Journal of Youth and Adolescence (1987), Special Issue on Sex and Gender Issues.

Keller, E. F. (1982), Feminism and science. *Signs*, 7:589–602.

——— (1983), Women, science, and popular mythology. In: *Machina Ex Dea*, ed. J. Rothschild. New York: Pergamon.

Kestenberg, J. S. (1968), Outside and inside, male and female. *J. Amer. Psychoanal. Assn.*, 16:457–520.

——— (1980), The inner genital phase. In: *Early Feminine Development: Contemporary Psychoanalytic Views*, ed. D. Mendel. New York: Spectrum, pp. 81–125.

Kirkpatrick, M., Ed. (1980), *Women's Sexual Development: Explorations of Inner Space*. New York: Plenum.

———— Ed. (1981), *Women's Sexual Experience: Explorations of the Dark Continent*. New York: Plenum.

Kleeman, J. A. (1965), A boy discovers his penis. *The Psychoanalytic Study of the Child*, 20:239–266. New York: International Universities Press.

———— (1966), Genital self-discovery during a boy's second year: A follow up. *The Psychoanalytic Study of the Child*, 21:358–392. New York: International Universities Press.

———— (1972), The establishment of core gender identity in normal girls. *Arch. Sex Behav.* 1:117–129.

Kohut, H. (1971), *The Analysis of the Self*. New York: International Universities Press.

Kubie, L. (1974), The drive to become both sexes. *Psychoanal. Quart.*, 43:349–426.

Lamb, M. E. (1976), *The Role of the Father in Child Development*. New York: John Wiley.

Laufer, M. (1976), The central masturbation fantasy, the final sexual organ, and adolescence. *The Psychoanalytic Study of the Child*, 31:297–316. New Haven, CT: Yale University Press.

Levin, M. (1988), Caring new world: Feminism and science. *Amer. Scholar*, 57:100–106.

Levinson, D., Darrow, C., Klein, E., Levinson, & McKee, B. (1978), *The Seasons of a Man's Life*. New York: Ballantine.

McDermott, J. F., Waldron, J. A., Char, W. F., Ching, J., Izatsu, S., Mann, E., Ponce, D. E., & Fukuanga, C. (1987), New female perceptions of power. *Amer. J. Psychiatry*. 144:1086–1087.

MacLusky, N. J., & Naftolin, F. (1981), Sexual differentiation of the central nervous system. *Science*, 211:1294–1303.

Mahfouz, A. M., & Smith, J. H. (1994), Introduction. In: *Psychoanalysis, Feminism, and the Future of Gender*, ed. A. M. Mahfouz & J. H. Smith. Baltimore: Johns Hopkins University Press, pp. ix–xv.

Mahler, M. (1969), *On Human Symbiosis and the Vicissitudes of Individuation*. Vol. 1. New York: International Universities Press.

———— Pine, F., & Bergman, A. (1975), *The Psychological Birth of the Human Infant*. New York: Basic Books.

Martin, A. D. (1982), Learning to hide: The socialization of the gay adolescent. *Adol. Psychiatry*, 10:52–65. Chicago: University of Chicago Press.

Mayer, E. L. (1995), The phallic castration complex and primary femininity: Paired developmental lines toward female gender identity. *J. Amer. Psychoanal. Assn.*, 43:17–38.

Meilhac, H., & Halevy, L. (1875), *Carmen, Libretto for Georges Bizet's Opera after Prosper Merimee's Novel*, tr. F. Merkling. Melville, NY: Belwin Mills, 1952.

Meyer, J. K. (1982), The theory of gender identity disorders. *J. Amer. Psychoanal. Assn.*, 30:381–418.

Michael, R. T., Gagnon, J. H., Laumann, E. O., & Kolata, G. (1994), *Sex in America*. Boston: Little, Brown.

Monette, P. (1992), *On Becoming a Man*. San Francisco: HarperCollins.

Money, J., & Ehrhardt, A. (1972), *Man and Woman, Boy and Girl*. Baltimore: Johns Hopkins University Press.

Morrison, N. K., & Severino, S. K. (1977), Moral influences: Development and gender influences. *J. Amer. Acad. Psychoanal.*, 25:255–277.

Offer, D., & Offer, J. B. (1975), *From Teenage to Young Manhood*. New York: Basic Books.

Panel (1987), Psychoanalysis of the young adult: Theory and technique. Reporter: J. F. Chused. *J. Amer. Psychoanal. Assn.*, 35:175–188.

Pratt, D. (1960), The Don Juan myth. *Amer. Imago*, 17:321–335.

Reich, H. (1960), *Children and Their Fathers*. New York: Hill & Wang.

Reiner, W. (1997), Editorial. To be male or female—that is the question. *Arch. Pediatr. Adolesc. Med.*, 151:224–225.

Rocah, B. (1989), Discussion of N. Chodorow's paper. *The Annual of Psychoanalysis*, 17:242–251. Hillsdale, NJ: Analytic Press.

Roiphe, H. (1968), On an early genital phase: With an addendum on genesis. *The Psychoanalytic Study of the Child*, 23:348–365. New York: International Universities Press.

——— Galenson, E. (1981), *Infantile Origins of Sexual Identities*. New York: International Universities Press.

Ross, J. M. (1975), The development of paternal identity: A critical review of the literature on nurturance and generativity in boys and men. *J. Amer. Psychoanal. Assn.*, 23:783–818.

——— (1983), Father to the child: Psychoanalytic reflections. *Psychoanal. Rev.*, 70:301–320.

Sayers, J. (1986), *Sexual Contradictions, Psychology, Psychoanalysis, and Feminism*. New York: Tavistock.

Schilder, P. (1938), *The Image and Appearance of the Human Body*. New York: International Universities Press, 1950.

Schneider, M. (1989), Sappho was a right-on adolescent: Growing up lesbian. In: *Gay And Lesbian Youth*, ed. G. Herdt. Binghamton, NY: Harrington Park Press, pp. 111–130.

Sherfey, M. J. (1966), Evolution and nature of female sexuality: Relation to psychoanalytic theory, *J. Amer. Psychoanal. Assn.*, 14:28–128.

Simmel, G. (1984), *On Women, Sexuality and Love*, tr. G. Oakes. New Haven, CT: Yale University Press.

Slipp, S. (1993), *The Freudian Mystique: Freud, Women, and Feminism*. New York: New York University Press.

Steinberg, L. (1987), Recent research on the family at adolescence: The extent and nature of sex differences. *J. Youth & Adol.*, 16:191–197.

Strouse, J. (1974), *Women and Analysis: Dialogues of Psychoanalytic Views of Femininity*, ed. J. Strouse. New York: Grossman.

Stoller, R. (1966), The mother's contribution to infantile transvestite behavior. *Internat. J. Psycho-Anal.*, 47:384–395.

——— (1968a), A further contribution to the study of gender identity. *Internat. J. Psycho-Anal.*, 49:364–367.

——— (1968b), *Sex and Gender*, Vol. 1. New York: Science House.

——— (1985), *Presentations of Gender*. New Haven, CT: Yale University Press.

Troiden, R. R. (1989), The formation of homosexual identities. In: *Gay and Lesbian Youth*, ed. G. Herdt. Binghampton, NY: Harrington Press, pp. 43–73.

Tyson, P. (1982), A developmental line for gender identity, gender role, and choice of love object. *J. Amer. Psychoanal. Assn.*, 30:61–86.

——— (1986a), Male gender identity: Early developmental roots. *Psychoanal. Rev.*, 73:405–425.

——— (1986b), Female psychological development as relived in the interaction between patient and analyst. Paper presented at a meeting of the Chicago Psychoanalytic Society, March.

——— (1986c), Female psychological development. *The Annual of Psychoanalysis*, 14:357–374. Hillsdale, NJ: Analytic Press.

——— (1989), Infantile sexuality, gender identity, obstacles in oedipal progress. *J. Amer. Psychoanal. Assn.*, 37:1049–1068.

——— (1994), Bedrock and beyond: An examination of the clinical utility of contemporary theories of female psychology. *J. Amer. Psychoanal. Assn.*, 42:447–467.

——— (1998), The psychology of women, continued. *J. Amer. Psychoanal. Assn.*, 46:361–363.

Vaillant, G. E. (1977), *Adaptation to Life*. Boston: Little, Brown.

Weissman, P. (1963), The effects of paternal attitudes on development and character. *Internat. J. Psycho-Anal.*, 44:121–131.

Wolf, E., & Wolf, I. (1979), We perished, each alone. A psychoanalytic commentary on Virginia Woolf's *To the Lighthouse*. *Internat. Rev. Psychoanal.*, 6:37–47.

Woolf, V. (1927), *To the Lighthouse*, New York: Harcourt, Brace.

Zucker, K. J., & Bradley, S. J. (1995), *Gender Identity Disorder and Psychosexual Problems in Children and Adolescents*. New York: Guilford Press.

Chapter 4

Intimacy

Erikson's concept of the normative developmental task of achieving intimacy versus isolation (1950, p. 229), is not limited to a sexual relationship. In addition, it refers to all those capacities of young adults for emotional closeness, trusting self-disclosure, mutual respect, joint problem solving, lessening ambivalence for the love object, and giving that person sufficient room to develop his or her potentials to the fullest. It also refers to sharing and resonating harmoniously with each other's deepest emotions of joy and sorrow and not engaging in destructive draining of the loved person's sharing of themselves. It is, in short, a relatively unambivalent relationship involving mutual love. Erikson's statement that young adults achieve intimacy only after they "emerge from their identity struggles" (p. 229) seems valid enough. Although, in-depth clinical observations would suggest that intimacy achievement simultaneously occurs alongside identity formation, and that the two tasks are the most important phase specific developmental tasks that young adult people are confronted with. In young adulthood, as well as throughout childhood and adolescence, there are different forms of intimacy with parents, siblings, friends, and peers.

Intimacy includes many different experiences: tenderness, gentleness, kindness, respect, friendship, nurturing, and being nurtured in an interdependency, collaboration, caring affection, romantic love, and not the least of all, sexuality. Both partners learn about the other's inner resources and vulnerabilities; what is offered, demanded, and withheld; and transformations of narcissism (Kohut, 1966). These ideal goals are part of the task of the late adolescent in his or her passage to young adulthood. The loving wife helps her husband realize his dream by believing in him and confirming his evolving identity. She acts as "teacher, guide, host, critic, [and] sponsor" (Levinson, Darrow, Klein, Levinson, and McKee, 1978, p. 109). The ideal loving husband reciprocates by being very supportive of his wife's dream in her career and as wife and mother. In fact, there are many recent instances of the husband (Mr. Mom) staying home with the children while his wife resumes her education and obtains a degree. Both partners have dreams that are heroic in nature, and the caring husband must nurture his wife's dream. As the young adult man learns to accept the feminine in himself and in others, he relaxes and learns to integrate a variety of feminine identifications. He learns that sharing household tasks and caring for children do not make him any less masculine. Instead, his marriage is strengthened, the children flourish, and he feels more committed. In addition, children thrive as a result of this greater exposure to their young adult father, because of a more balanced environment.

On the other hand, untransformed narcissistic needs exist in those individuals who force intimacy on spouses, children, and employees. Sexually, verbally, or physically victimized children and spouses often feel obligated to remain attached because of an overpowering fear of abandonment. It seems that there is a connection between gender and readiness for parenthood. The young college women in Litwak's (1985) study, were often afraid of the dangers of intimacy, and specifically of the risks of being hurt. Their capacities to cope are tied to the level of ego development and their fears of dependency. All the women in this study were of superior intellect as measured by grade point averages. Overall, however, most young women are somewhat more ready for and competent with this developmental step than are young adult men, since they achieve this capacity for intimacy earlier by a few years. Young men are primarily concerned with getting established in their careers and consolidating their vocational identity. In addition, young men are quite concerned about solidifying their sexual competence before taking on the responsibility of children. It was in this context that Erikson paraphrased Freud's concept of genitality in terms of the capacity for love and work (1950, p. 229). To be sure intimacy is integrally connected to the sexual drive in both men and women and is experienced in both as a desire for closeness, but in women it is most often directly connected to fantasies and dreams of realizing procreative aims. Some modern women may, however, merely seek closeness and intimacy without significant conscious or unconscious desires for parenthood. Young adult men for the most part are regularly concerned with fears of entrapment and of being dominated or controlled by women who are unconsciously perceived in fantasy as the phallic castrating or omnipotent, destructive, enveloping, and intrusive maternal object.

Gabriel (1987) reported that a growing number of American men voiced their fears ("it's scary," p. 24) of getting married. The latest census data quoted in this article document that 13.8 percent of 30- to 44-year-old men have never married, an increase of 9 percent from the previous decade. The most common stated fear was one of entrapment, even though they admire those men who have made a commitment to a woman and have children. One person quoted said that he felt "relationships always seemed very stifling. They [women] change your life around and don't allow you a lot of freedom to roam. Not roam to pick up women. Just roam to do stuff" (p. 32). Some men also seem to be holding out for the perfect woman. Gabriel postulates that women suspect men to be Don Juanlike characters, but the men he interviewed didn't fit that classical description. Instead, what he discovered was that "many men, frankly, seemed to be withdrawing from particularly active sex lives" (p. 32). He feels AIDS is a factor, but more importantly men are retreating from the sexual revolution that characterized the 1960s. What these men are engaged in now are sports and building up their bodies. One of the men interviewed saw himself as a protracted adolescent like the poet Yeats who remained a bachelor well into adulthood. It was as though the excitement of the pursuit of women for sex alone had diminished to the point of extinction of the stimulus. Women suspect that men are more interested in sexual conquests than in establishing a permanent intimate relationship. "Either he is a Don Juanish character whose ego needs the continuous reinforcement of new conquests, or, perhaps he needs to confuse sex with intimacy" (p. 32). One man has discovered from his sample of about 300 women he has dated that many are quite cold and very satisfied with remaining single to pursue a career.

A sociological study by Lynn Jamieson (1998), Senior Lecturer at the University of Edinburgh, suggests that equality between the sexes has not reached parity as yet in parenting and domestic chores. She found that the more employment-oriented partner distances himself or herself from those activities. In fact, it looks like a major shift toward greater intimacy in present Western culture has not yet occurred. In fact, intimacy is much more of a theoretical ideal since large numbers of the population of Western industrialized nations seem to be more interested in self-fulfillment and autonomy.

Masturbation fantasies held over from adolescence influence the developing and unfolding sexuality of the young adult. In this regard, Ritvo (cited in Panel, 1987) and Laufer (1976) believe that unique adolescent masturbatory fantasies influence the shaping of adult sexuality in both men and women. Pathologically, there may be some holdover from adolescence of guilt, phobic anxiety, and mystification about sexual fantasies or activity with a partner. This complicates settling down permanently with one partner. In fact, some men experience commitment to another person as too restraining and clearly are not ready for an intimate relationship. An example of this problem of intimacy was contrasted with Larry's rise in business. It was meteoric, but he resisted making a permanent commitment to a young woman with whom he was deeply in love. He was puzzled about his reluctance to make a commitment. What restrained him, we discovered, were unconscious resentments toward his mother for divorcing his father, and much earlier for replacing him with his two younger siblings. Guilt over competitive strivings with his father were only a small part of these dynamics at this point. Competitiveness with his father was, in fact, sublimated into business activities and served to keep oedipal related strivings repressed in the dynamic unconscious.

In some heterosexual men wishes for closeness, moreover, become confused with fears of being homosexual, especially when there has been a history of open conflicts with father and frustrated regressive wishes for a passive reconciliation. A case in point was Robert, a 26-year-old lawyer, whose father had died two years earlier. Robert had started drinking early in adolescence, graduated to drugs soon thereafter in an angry rebellion against the loss of a loving close relative and the fact that his father was always too busy with his professional life to devote any time to him. While he wished for a greater degree of emotional intimacy with his wife, he was consumed with regressive sexual fantasies. The fact that he couldn't accomplish the task of adult intimacy pained him deeply. The analysis uncovered the unconscious reason for these feelings. It was a towering rage against his father, which was being displaced onto his wife and various other individuals. The transference was maintained at an optimal level by carefully timed and

phrased interpretations in keeping with Chused's (1987) rec-
ommendation that idealization of the therapist is essential for
the resolution of negative oedipal conflicts in young adult men.

Certain pathological narcissistic "attitudes of entitlement
and spurious autonomy" (Rodgers, 1991) are still another
source of interference with establishing intimacy in young
adults. Some young adult married couples get caught up in
neurotic interactions stemming from narcissistically distorted
self and self–selfobject representations that unconsciously interfere with a healthy deepening of intimacy. For example, one
young man continued a pattern into young adulthood that had
begun much earlier in adolescence. Often, he would launch a
home improvement project to gain his father's approval, but
invariably his father would unempathically criticize and humili-
ate his son. This set up a rageful enmity that could only be
resolved by the son tearfully retreating to his room, with his
father being made to feel guilty enough to come and console
the injured son. Often the father would ignore the imposition
of guilt, but when he did succumb to it, there was a mutually
heart-wrenching attempt at reconciliation. Most often, however, reconciliation misfired, because neither father nor son
was capable at the time of much emotional intimacy. They
avoided each other like the plague and were very estranged
when the analysis started in late adolescence. The father constantly belittled all his children as well as his wife. No one was
ever good enough for him. The patient felt closer to his
mother, but he could not respect her because of her passive
submission to the abusive father. He dated very little throughout high school and college because he was tense and uncom-
fortable with women. Much analytic work yielded insight into
the oedipal meaning of his conflict with his father as it was
reenacted in the transference which in turn led to a more
cordial nonconflictual relationship with his father. My patient
then gathered his courage to tentatively venture into a more

satisfying and intimate relationship with a suitable young woman.

In a relationship begun in early adolescence, Walter hoped to find the emotional intimacy of a family that he had never experienced. Susan's mother proceeded to relive her own adolescence by openly competing with her daughter in thinly disguised sexual overtures and gestures. These triadic interactions were poorly and inadequately processed by both husband and wife. As long as the wife felt she was winning the struggle by a comfortable margin, she was able to tolerate the anxiety generated by these incestuous games. In addition, his mother fought to hold onto her son by every means possible. For example, she would call him up during each date, requesting that he bring her a newspaper, and in effect beg him to come home to her. When the wife was confronted with a real rival, however, she succumbed to regressive infantile tantrums, demanding to be taken on trips and other tangible proofs and reassurances of a secure hold on him. Intimacy, however, still suffered because of a serious sexual inhibition.

Mary was a 21-year-old school teacher who arrived for her first appointment accompanied by her mother. She was engaged to be married, but was plagued by many fears. She was frightened of traveling alone into the city from the suburbs. Her fiancé was especially sensitive to her fears and did not become exasperated with her. He was patient with her fears of sexual intimacy and did not demand more than she could tolerate. Additionally, she suffered from a form of vaginal spasm that had to be dilated by the gynecologist. When her concerns about separation from her mother, who was reluctant to let her daughter leave home, were sufficiently brought to consciousness and worked through, she married and subsequently had several children.

A 30-year-old female graduate student in music had returned to music as a career five years after pursuing a career in another field. She was acutely and severely depressed. She was phobic and obsessively worried about a nuclear war and afraid of getting involved in a relationship after the breakup of a passionate relationship with another musician who was emotionally and otherwise unavailable. She was enormously affected by her parents' views and opinions and was afraid she would submit wholesale to their expected urgings to leave treatment just as she was getting better. The transference took shape in the form of expecting the analyst to be as intrusive and critically deflating as her parents had been, especially her mother. Her weakened and fragile self was gradually strengthened when she was able to internalize her experiences in the new transference relationship with the analyst who carefully helped her to establish her own boundaries.

SUMMARY

Finally, it is clear from these brief clinical vignettes that intimacy and identity formation proceed together to form the process of transition to young adulthood, though in practice too many people are so self absorbed as to prevent themselves from ever developing real intimacy with a suitable partner. Like Erikson (1950), Marcia (1980) considered that intimacy is the heir of identity formation.

What has been implied by the foregoing clinical examples is that the capacity for intimacy emerges when an integration of the elements of identity formation, namely identification and socialization processes, construct a viable and enduring but evolving identity.

REFERENCES

Chused, J. F. (1987), Idealization of the analyst by the young adult. *J. Amer. Psychoanal. Assn.*, 35:839–859.

Erikson, E. H. (1950), *Childhood and Society*. New York: W. W. Norton.

Gabriel, T. (1987), Why wed?: The ambivalent bachelor. *NY Times Magazine*, 6:24–34; 60, November 15.

Jamieson, L. (1998), *Intimacy*. Cambridge, U.K.: Polity.

Kohut, H. (1966), Forms and transformations of narcissism. *J. Amer. Psychoanal. Assn.*, 14:243–272.

Laufer, M. (1976), The central masturbation fantasy, the final sexual organ, and adolescence. *The Psychoanalytic Study of the Child*, 31:297–316. New Haven, CT: Yale University Press.

Levinson, D. J., Darrow, C. N., Klein, E. B., Levinson, M. H., & McKee, B. (1978), *The Seasons of a Man's Life*. New York: Knopf.

Litwak, N. (1985), Fear of intimacy among college women. *Adol.*, 20:15–20.

Marcia, J. E. (1980), Identity in adolescence. In: *Handbook of Adolescent Psychology*, ed. J. Adelson. New York: John Wiley, pp. 159–187.

Panel (1987), Psychoanalysis of the young adult: Theory and technique. Reporter: J. F. Chused. *J. Amer. Psychoanal. Assn.*, 35:175–188.

Rodgers, T. C. (1991), Book review: *Narcissism and Intimacy: Love and Marriage in an Age of Confusion* by M. F. Solomon. *Psychoanal. Books*, 2:272–274. New York: W. W. Norton.

Chapter 5

The Fate of Don Juan: The Myth and the Man

> Nature has placed but one law in my bosom, to do
> nothing but what pleases me [Maetzu, 1938, p. 202].

This chapter will contain a discussion of late adolescent and young adult character development (Deutsch, 1965) in certain individuals whose behavior is reminiscent of the dramatic and mythic character of Don Juan Tenorio, whose motives for control and power over others, as manifest in his sexual exploits, are legendary (e.g., Mozart's opera *Don Giovanni*). The three important motivations of late adolescence, mastery of sexuality, acquisition of power over others, and interest in accumulating money, certainly flower in adolescence and young adulthood. Motives such as these are less obvious than the externally more visible pubertal and maturational (physiological) changes of adolescence or the cognitive and intellectual changes, but they are nevertheless very important. Of these three, power and control or dominance over others have been sorely neglected in recent psychoanalytic literature.

A previous version of this chapter under the same title was published in *Adolescent Psychiatry* (1992), 18:44–62. It is reprinted by permission of University of Chicago Press.

117

Fenichel (1945, pp. 243–244) discusses these motivations in terms of libido theory and infantile sexuality, specifically in the anal phase, or sadism and omnipotence. The "Oedipal complex is dominated by the pregenital aim of incorporation, pervaded by narcissistic needs and tinged with sadistic impulses" (p. 243). Horner (1989) claims that the power of self arises as a mastery over childhood helplessness and powerlessness and is commonly repeated in adolescence in relation to parental control (see also chapter 6).

Before describing any of the clinical phenomena, it seems appropriate to review the story of the classical figure of Don Juan. The original play, one of more than three hundred, was written by Tirso de Molina (Fra Gabriel Tellez, a Mercerdarian monk) in the early part of the seventeenth century during the golden age of Spanish drama, and published in 1630 (Flores, 1991). His mentor was the great dramatist Lope de Vega. It is interesting to note that Tirso de Molina was in his early twenties at the time he wrote this play. Tirso was born of unknown parents in Madrid around 1583 and lived in Toledo from 1605 to 1615, a decade of the greatest literary exuberance. "Tirso's keen insight and sense of comedy..." (Kunitz and Colby, 1967, pp. 645–646) are represented in his other plays, but it is in his *El Burlador* that "Don Juan is a vital incarnation of sensuality, endlessly devoted to the pursuit of pleasure" (Kunitz and Colby, 1967, p. 646). Havelock Ellis (1908) commented that Tirso's Don Juan and his flaming passion are melded in the Spanish character with the passionate ascetic mysticism of Saint Teresa of Avila.

The original title of the play is *El Burlador de Sevilla y Convividado de Piedra*, "The Jester of Seville and the Stone Guest." *Burlador* has been translated as "Jester" but other meanings are "Rake," "Joker," "Trickster," "Rogue," "Prankster," "Seducer," "Playboy" (Mandel, 1963), or "Mocker," all of which convey some part of the meaning. *Trickster* is the most commonly used term in the literature.

Don Juan is depicted as a late adolescent visiting his uncle, the Spanish ambassador to the king of Naples. He makes love to a series of women, beginning with the Duchess Isabella, who is betrothed to Don Octavio, and then back in Spain, Dona Ana, who is betrothed to the Marquis de la Mota. Dona Ana's father, Don Gonzalo de Ulloa, is the Commendatore of the Order of Calatrava, and is killed by Don Juan in the act of defending his daughter's honor. In addition, there are two peasant girls who are seduced in the play.

An essential feature of Don Juan's seductions involves stealing women away from their betrothed, or in one case (Tisbea), a determined state of virginity, and then tricking the women into having sex with him. Don Juan is quite creative in devising successful tactics that he tailors for each seduction. The second part of the story, which Tirso de Molina brilliantly merges with the sexual exploits of Don Juan, concerns his mocking invitation to the stone statue of the Commendatore to dine with him. The Commendatore agrees only if his slayer returns the favor. In the end, *El Burlador* is carried off to hell in retribution for his sins, capping what is distinctly a morality play. Besides being entertaining, this play was very likely designed to frighten off would-be imitators of Don Juan's lifestyle with eternal punishment. The rebellious, willful, late adolescent behavior of Don Juan in the play brings consternation and exasperation to his father and the king of Seville, a story familiar to modern parents. But what is most striking is the fact that his mother is never mentioned.

The term *legendary* is merely descriptive, for Don Juan was, of course, a mythic character (Worthington, 1962) not a living person. The play was probably based on earlier Spanish stories extant in the culture of seventeenth-century Spain (D. McClelland, 1975). In the eighteenth century a real person named

Don Miguel de Manara imitated Don Juan''s lifestyle only to repent later, and become an ascetic. He donated all his money to build a children's hospital in Seville.

It is interesting to read Hume's (1927) historical reconstruction from primary sources about the court of Philip IV, the "Planet King"—"that monarch with the long tragic uncanny face, whose impassive mask and raging soul within" . . . (as painted by Velasquez) presided over the fall of the great Spanish Empire. He and his wife Isabel loved the theater and when he attended the theater he sat behind a grill or latticework incognito wearing a mask, since the king was not supposed to be seen at such vulgar entertainments. However, he had a private entrance with access to the actresses on stage. The women spectators sat separately in a *cazuela* where the king could look them over for possible new conquests. Philip also used the theater to see his various mistresses. In fact, he was a veritable Don Juan himself, once almost consummating an affair with a beautiful nun, and fathering some thirty or forty illegitimate children. His favorite and chief minister, Count Olivares, kept him supplied with women and as well put on frequent costume balls and parades. The king himself wrote plays and he would "frequently propos[e] a subject for an impromptu play in the facile blank verse which comes so tripplingly upon the Spanish lips. The subject would sometimes be a sacred one, in which case the treatment was such as would shock modern ears . . ." (Hume, 1927, pp. 200–201). The theaters Corral de la Pacheca and Corral de la Cruz were crowded every day, "the plays presented, hundreds of which are still extant, are marvelous in the inventive fertility of their plots, the intrigues that spring from mistaken personality, marital wiles, and lovers' stratagems furnishing the foundation of most of them" (Hume, 1927, p. 202). Several grandees were banished for scaling the walls of the Bien Retiro palace to make love to the maids of honor.

The Countess Danois (1774), whether the name of a real person or a pseudonym, wrote in a series of letters about her observations of Philip IV, his court, and the culture of the time. She particularly noted the spendthrift government that squandered the riches derived from the Americas, and those elements of the character of Spanish men of the time that resembled the mythic Don Juan Tenorio, and the women who to some extent allowed themselves to be seduced.

The uncompromising outcome that was Don Juan's fate in the play has been surprisingly neglected in psychoanalytic interpretations of the myth, except in the seminal work of Otto Rank (1924). Tirso de Molina's extraordinary plot has spawned many versions of the original story, including those by Moliere, Byron, Shaw, Shadwell, Manara, Kierkegaard, Dumas, Maranon, Walcott, Zorilla, Tolstoy, and Camus among others, but many of these authors diluted the essential character of Don Juan and turned him into a withered old man, an absurd hero (as in Camus' work [Weinstein, 1967]) or a bland character not at all interested in sex (as in Shaw's *Man and Superman*, 1903; Mandel, 1963). On the other hand, Richard Strauss and Mozart composed musical masterpieces around the theme of a proud and brave nobleman whose sole aim in life is short-term selfish pleasure (Maetzu, 1938). The original play depicts Don Juan as a very erotic character who lives to make love, and, interestingly enough, women are delighted with his prowess and are willing partners. The popular appeal of both the play and Mozart's opera, as well as Strauss's tone poem, shows that the idealization of exuberant late adolescent sexuality is a constant theme over hundreds of years.

The case material of a clinical psychoanalysis presented in this chapter displays the central core clinical problem around issues of control, subjugation of others, or dominance in the transference situation that had multiple conscious and unconscious manifestations and meanings. For example, there were recurrent struggles over the appointment schedule and resistance to the process of free association. Furthermore, it was equally true in the real relationships with women as it was in the transference situation. A more detailed description follows, but suffice it to say control by subjugation was the paradigmatic defense transference. Winter (1973) has suggested a defense deployed against the "chaos and confusion of incorporation." In a way, this is correct, but a more precise interpretation refers to certain control measures that are deployed against the loss or threatened rupture in the idealized and fused relationship with the internal image of the mother. In the transference, my patient was threatened with feelings of abandonment over weekends and vacations. He usually went into a rage and demanded his way about the most mundane of issues. Motives for dominating control, subjugation and power over others are seen as originating in early childhood, and these issues later on merge with adolescent phallic aggressiveness, sexualization, and exhibitionism in the form of a display of cavalier seduction of any and all those women the Don Juan character perceives as a challenge.

The motive for dominating control and power over others in group processes (Fenichel, 1945, pp. 502–504) may emerge from similar sources, but group processes are much more complicated and deserve a separate study. I would only say at this time that exhibitionism and the love of power for its own sake and aggressivization take the place of sexualization processes. There is a very strong sense of neediness. Fenichel also suggested that the desire for power may be derived from anal sadism and mastery of sphincter control (p. 283), or a defense against deep-seated or archaic anxieties about oral conflicts (p. 479). Fenichel's formulation is that the Oedipus complex is distorted wherein sexual strivings are "condensed with the strivings for narcissistic supplies in order to maintain self-esteem" (p. 243).

To return to dominating sexual motivations, I would like to say that it seems reasonable to assume that various forms of hypersexuality occur along a continuum, at one end of which is the Don Juan (or Casanova) complex (Trachtenberg, 1988), nymphomania, certain instances of homosexual behavior, and use of multiple partners in both heterosexuals and homosexuals. At the other end, are the phase-appropriate experimental efforts in adolescence on the way to adulthood to master and integrate sexuality. By this I mean those tasks of adolescence, as originally stated by Erikson (1959), to relish and integrate and not just tolerate intimacy with one person with whom a permanent commitment is made. Also, during adolescence fantasies of living out a Don Juan lifestyle are very common and probably serve very important and constructively adaptive purposes. Don Juan derives the use of power from his pursuit of pleasure of the moment, while punishment by death is far away (*Tan largo me fiais*). He is creatively resourceful in using every trick in his bag of seduction games (Maetzu, 1938) to accomplish his arrogant excesses. Through his rebellious defiance of the everlasting, his father, and the king, and his extraordinary vitality, creativity, sensuality, arrogant courage, and humor, Don Juan in general expresses in the play "man's challenge to the world of his limitations" (I. L. McClelland, 1967, p. 586). "The power of this drama derives from its rapid pace, the impression it gives of cumulative tension as Don Juan's enemies gradually hound him to destruction, and the electrifying fact that he is goaded by excess to defy, beyond redeemable limits, even the ghostly forces of the unknown. Refusing to repent he crashes to eternal damnation" (I. L. McClelland, 1967, p. 586). Don Juan is looking for an ideal woman but not for real love because he is a selfish romantic whose grandiosity includes the belief that not a single woman in the world is worthy of him. He doesn't love any woman as much as he would like to be loved. He is not in love and yet his extraordinary sensuality, egotistical pride, and courage account for his power. He is without a doubt crudely resourceful, using any trick that works to complete a seduction. He has no ideals, just pure sensuality without regard for morality. What else does one need, he says, when one has had a woman, good food, mellow evenings, and a good wine. Don Juan is irrepressibly bigger than life; he fears "nothing, trusting nothing but his valor and his sword . . . [and] in his veins surges the blood of those grandees who have made and unmade both priests and kings. In him is the spirit of those proud beings who disdained the easy servitude of the moorish invaders, of those conquistadores who ventured the perils of the unknown seas to win the fabled wealth of the Indes" (Austen, 1939, pp. 340–341).

If he were more humanly flexible or subject to change, he would, like my patient, eventually fall for a woman. So in a way the secret to the fascination in the play is Don Juan's never ending energy and the fact that he never falls in love with a woman. "He is a fantasy with absolute power and freedom imposing his will over women. He is the incarnation of free will" (Maetzu, 1938, p. 89).[1] For him, it is no sin to kill or seduce women, but his right.

However, as interesting as the literary character is, it is important at this point to differentiate the literary character from the clinically observed person since the literary Don Juan is an imaginary person in whom certain humanlike qualities are highlighted and exaggerated in the play and these qualities are not necessarily present in the same combinations in real human beings.

Anecdotally, Anais Nin described both her father and an opera singer friend, whom she called Siegfried, as Don Juan characters. She understood the typical Don Juan to be a charmingly lovable man who is attracted and devoted to women "always at the beginning, at the first moment of faith and love . . ."

---

[1]Translated by Pedro Jose Cevallos Candau.

(Nin, 1966-1971, p. 272) who never stays around to watch the relationship deteriorate. He is there only to satisfy his own pleasure. The renowned French mystery writer, Georges Simenon, claimed he had slept with ten thousand women and Simone de Beauvoir (1985) described Jean-Paul Satre's many sexual adventures as similar to Don Juan's. The female (Dona Juana) and some homosexual counterparts present some interesting differences, but the essential quality of unbridled sensuality remains the same, and a similar formulation to the one presented here seems adequate to explain the phenomenon.

CLINICAL EXAMPLE

While the outcome of adolescent character development is hard to predict during adolescence, studying the process of development retrospectively presents much less of a problem and is typically part of good clinical work, as Freud pointed out (1920) early on. The following is a condensation of an analysis that suffers from the distortions of efforts to distill the essence of certain pathological character formations and specific defenses encountered.

   Mr. H was 40 years old, divorced, and a professional man. He came for analysis with symptoms of a long-standing depression, inability to form a lasting and loving relationship with a woman, intense anxieties, and ruminative concerns about his erratic business successes and failures. He looked and behaved like a much younger man. He had trouble going to sleep and staying asleep. He was a handsome man with a swarthy complexion, slight in build, but very muscular. Superficially, he was assertive and forthcoming so that it was easy to see that he was attractive to women. He smoked too much and life held too few pleasures. His past history revealed a Don Juan-type character beginning in adolescence. He claimed he had relationships with some forty or fifty women with whom he had brief encounters. He had been married briefly in his twenties, but that marriage had ended in divorce. He had achieved some progress in a previous therapy, finishing a graduate degree in business and achieving some partial stability in his private and business life. However, this therapy had reached a stalemate, and he had reluctantly and ambivalently terminated it.

As we began our work together, it was apparent early on that his chief concern was his inability to effect a close relationship with a suitable woman. In spite of many sexual successes, he was tired of the emptiness and loneliness of a life that no longer brought much excitement or delight in the conquests.

After an extended diagnostic period, we decided on psychoanalysis as the treatment of choice. Very soon thereafter, he initiated a relationship with a woman. The death knell for the Don Juan behavior, however, had sounded some time before, when the underlying depression had surfaced.

What follows is a more detailed account of the middle phase of the analysis, beginning about a year after we started. He was angry when he felt controlled and manipulated by his woman friend. "She tries to make me into something I'm not. I told her I thought she was very demanding. She fights me on every point. I can't see why because other women give me my way." He was frustrated and angry when his most minute demands were not met. Similarly, he fantasized about getting control over me in the transference regarding appointment times and questioned me extensively about the analytic process, but then he became fearful that I would not like him and he regressed to wanting to be coddled and comforted. He recalled that his mother overdid coddling, and we constructed a confining early childhood situation. What frequently followed was a grandiose fantasy that he could surely please me by performing extraordinary business-related tasks and making a lot of money, but he was overcome in the transference with fear that I would be like

God who would "punish me and take it all away." Typically, during this period, interpretations were made to clarify what I thought to be the central transference meanings of the clinical data. For example, I pointed out his fears of competition in his business ventures, in his relationships with women, and particularly with me in the father transference. These interpretations had little or no effect on the transference or his symptoms.

Then his mother died unexpectedly. Right away, the character of the analysis came under the sway of the mourning process. He was unable to mourn at first. He said, "I can't cry. There just aren't any tears and besides I have to keep up appearances for my father's sake." He dreamed of having sex with a man, moving in with his father, and in fantasy getting his mother's ring. He has always wanted to be a star for his father and now me in the transference. Accepting defeat, though, invariably led to symptoms of depression and self-defeating behavior. In a dream precipitated by a separation from me, he was afraid I would be angry that he was abandoning me. He acted out by performing many of his mother's domestic tasks for his father. The negative oedipal interpretation of these dynamics seemed cogent at the time, but as the analysis proceeded and deepened an entirely different picture emerged.

As he momentarily regained control over these regressive unconscious wishes to replace his mother, he contacted a previous girl friend who readily responded to his every whim. "What I enjoy is the power of that experience." What he meant was that this woman was passively submissive and was content to satisfy his every need. After having sex, he would send her home in a cab. He fantasized about marrying a totally subjugated oriental woman who would follow him around and cater to him. It gave him a powerful sense of dominating control. Physical tension was released by similar brief sexual encounters during which he was in complete control. However, he was more strongly drawn to women who physically and character- ologically resembled his mother, that is, women who were pe- tite but intrusive and reluctant to permit separations.

Each separation, whether generated by him or by me, led to feelings of angry helplessness, anxious depression, and loss of sufficient energies to do his work—in a word, he collapsed. When his girl friend obtained a divorce, he felt pressure from her to make a commitment. During his marriage and again now, he felt taken over and controlled by a close relationship that demanded greater intimacy. These demands encroached on a hard-won equilibrium consisting of his private free time to watch his favorite television shows and go to bed early. He claimed he needed much rest from the frenzy of his daily striv- ings, through which he hoped to impress his father and me in the idealizing transference. He was envious and angry with other patients, whom he felt got preferential treatment from me. This was interpreted to mean that he felt I was indifferent to his particular needs like his father had been.

Paradoxically, after major losses of income, it seemed that his head was clearer and he was able to pull himself together enough to recover some of his losses. Analysis of this paradox brought out a restitutional fantasy that he needed sympathy from me similar to what he had invariably gotten from his father to alleviate the shame and guilt of his failures. He dreamed of feeling strong enough to confront me as a belliger- ent adversary, but at the last minute stepped aside and excused himself. Abortive attempts at self-assertion, however, were in- frequent. He was desperate to be a star for me. He discussed in detail his business problems, hoping to get some secret clue about his failures, but this invariably led to feelings of shame, despair, and defeat. This depressing cycle was deepened and further complicated by a sleep disorder.

Feeling as if he were second best made him very angry. As he ruminated about these feelings, he got more angry and more depressed. He hated himself and his failures to meet his grandiose goals. In his own words, "I'm always trying to hit a home run instead of just making dimes. I should be more aggressive without being wild and taking too big a risk. It's so sad that my father will die some day and I've never succeeded for him. It's more sad for him now that mother is gone."

He described the symptomatic onset of his neurosis seven or eight years earlier. He saw women less frequently, and with only one or two would he have brief sexual encounters. There was no sense of permanence or stability. He no longer went prowling with his sidekick (his version of Catalinon or Leporello). As noted, it was as if the adolescent behavior pattern began to deteriorate and be replaced by a serious depression. He used to be more energetic in a regular sport activity in which he had to have the ball all the time. A little later on in the treatment, he felt more confident to reveal other details of his neurosis, namely, that he was nervous in large crowds.

> It has always been that way. I don't like to go out to parties and dress up, put on a suit and a tie. That's why I wear casual clothes all the time because I feel very shy and insecure. I think it all started when my father [repeatedly] told me I was second best. I've spent my whole life feeling inferior. In college, people called me humiliating nicknames. That's when I started to smoke. This is another reason why I need a lot of rest. I started to take a lot of drugs and went to Europe for four months. Now, when I'm attracted to women, I can't get close. I chase them away, and I can't keep involved. What I want the most is to be number one with my father [and me in the transference].

As the analysis proceeded into the third year, he continued to be preoccupied with feeling manipulated and dominated by women who demanded that he do their bidding; for example, as to when they made love or whether to dress up to go out to dinner. He doubted his future would be any better, and he was obsessively angry about every instance of perceived manipulation. He withheld his love unless he felt he had complete control. At this point, he announced that he was leaving for a three-week winter vacation with his father.

When he recalled a childhood image of himself as a passive, wimpy, unaggressive little boy, he thought that image was an attempt to comply with his parents' unempathic admonition that he behave more like a neighbor girl, as if to say "put on a dress." This and similar humiliations were frequent. In contrast to his internal image of himself, he was told he was hyperactive as a small child—a "wild Indian"—because all the precious objects in the house had to be put up out of his reach.

As the analytic work proceeded, he reported that he had been feeling stronger, taller, and more aggressive. In fact, he reported that he had a more financially successful year than previously. Telling me of his good fortune, however, was again followed by some costly business mistakes. He said, "Every time I reach for the stars, I come up with cobwebs." In a dream about his mother, the surface meaning was to replace his mother, but the deeper meaning involved a wish to reestablish a close relationship with me in the idealized mother transference. This was acted out when he talked on the telephone with his sister every day just as she had done with their mother before her death.

"In all the photos from my childhood, I'm on the outside next to my mother," the unconsciously preferred position. We reconstructed the early childhood experience of being overwhelmed with feelings of overstimulation and abandonment from his mother and humiliation from his father. Also, the father, who had lost a parent in childhood, was not around to help him separate from the mother. My patient missed his mother now and was for the first time deeply involved in the mourning process. A dream of looking for refuge from a storm revealed the transference meaning of expecting me, like mother, to magically relieve his distress, but he feared the worst. He was very sad and depressed, with no hope or prospect of recovery. He said, "Life has no meaning."

Another dream quickly followed with the similar meaning of being rescued but with an additional meaning of his fear of increasing involvement with women and me, as mother. In the idealized mother transference, he perceived me as forcing him into a helpless, submissive, and dependent but overstimulated relationship similar to what existed with his mother and from which he struggled to escape. He simultaneously feared and longed for this reunion with mother. As he prepared for another separation, he tried to minimize the disruption by shortening the time away. When he returned, he experienced another cycle of attempted closeness and withdrawal precipitated by his fears of being controlled and manipulated in the transference. He toyed with the idea of terminating therapy by talking about ending the relationship with his woman friend. He acted this out by reducing the frequency of the sessions as a way of restoring control over me in the analytic situation.

As though to calm himself about the increased tension in the analysis, he recalled how he was invariably successful in bar hopping with his buddy to pick up women. He believed he could never be the success that he thought his father or I demanded, or for that matter, acquire a healthy sense of self-worth. Fantasies of acquiring a family by marrying his woman friend (who had several lovely children) made him feel better because he expected that I (and his parents) would be pleased. In a romantic mood, he thought of giving her his mother's diamond ring. He dreamed of being very angry at me as his father for "busting my ass for him." He struggled to assert himself in the transference relationship by telling me off just before leaving for a vacation. These fantasies and efforts to assert himself were experimental efforts to move beyond the idealizing mother transference.

During the fourth year of the analysis, he began to feel more in control, and his image of himself improved significantly. He liked the image of being a family man and a father. There was no question that the woman friend was in love with him, though somewhat ambivalently and fearful of getting hurt. When she withdrew out of anxiety and dated other men, it made him crazy with jealousy. He felt abandoned. Demanding exclusive rights over her made her balk. In desperation, he proposed, but she said it was too early and played for time. It seemed to him that she was acting like an adolescent girl rebelling against her mother, who had forbidden her to see other men, and unwittingly he had fallen into the same trap. As a matter of fact, she enjoyed the attention of several men.

In more ways than one, he had met his match. One could say that she was a kind of Don Juana. With her behavior, she was declaring her independence from him and her mother. One way of looking at their relationship was that she and my patient were mirror images of each other.

When she went off for a weekend with other people he got a dose of his own medicine and as he put it, he went "bonkers"—he really couldn't stand being abandoned by her. He was terrified by the thought she was sleeping with other men. The sparks flew as they quarreled over who would control whom. He looked to me for direct advice on how to cope and solve such a dilemma of an impossible and uncontrollable woman. He was a very jealous lover who brooked no competition. He was frantic.

During the summer interruption in the analysis, both he and his woman friend became even more anxious about a permanent commitment to each other. This was followed by a brief interruption in the relationship. His response was that he felt he could not trust her. He felt betrayed and disillusioned. On one or two occasions, he even followed her around to spy on her actions. He again sank into a depression and felt himself to be a magnificent failure. In this state, he felt helpless and out of control. He repeated his demand for an exclusive relationship with her. Controlling her actions and wanting her to submit to his needs were clearly major motivations in this man. When control failed, he withdrew. The woman friend responded with an infantile neediness that made him feel he was being converted into her mother, especially when she wanted to talk on the phone late at night. He spitefully refused. As both of them calmed down from this lovers' quarrel, he feared he could never escape.

Just before another interruption in the analysis, he experienced an increase in anxiety and a mild roller coaster kind of excitement and depression. In a word, he was desperate to get something from me. Symptomatic of this state was the fact he couldn't stop his cigarette addiction. He had tried everything, including hypnotism and nicotine gum. He repeated that he considered himself a failure. He felt he couldn't control anything or anyone, including me in the transference. To say that the therapy was near another stalemate is too dramatic. At any rate, interpretations of the transference alone seemed to be insufficiently helpful.

At this point, I prescribed a mild sedative that facilitated regaining inner control. He slept better. The transference meaning of giving him something that he had not gotten from his father was made clear. He stopped smoking for good. While control and power issues remained important concerns and potential sources of conflict, he was much less consumed with them. He was more in control of his rages and was more trusting. When he returned from a winter vacation, power struggles with me and his woman friend had decreased significantly. Before, making love had been like possessing, dominating, and controlling her, but now there was more mutuality and trust.

In the transference, he was more trusting and collaborating. Before, when he felt he was losing control, he got angry and contentious, but now he was more serene and confident. These changes were due mainly to the analysis and only in a minor fashion resulted from the medication. After four months, we gradually reduced the medication without any retrogressive symptomatology.

I prefer to confine my presentation not to a single case to illustrate my thesis. Therefore, I should like to mention some other data. For example, women who display Don Juan behavior have been described by Kavesh and Lavin (1989). They referred to the type A woman who, though married, toys with the idea of having an affair. She is always on the lookout for men and misses the chase. One woman said she liked "the tension and excitement of an early romance. I haven't felt that with my husband since our son was born three years ago." Similarly, the beautiful but vindictive noblewoman in *Dangerous Liaisons* (derived from Laclos, 1782) is another analogous version of Don Juana. She wreaks vengeance on her unfaithful lover, the Viscount, who has spent his life seducing new virginal challenges. But he lost out in the end, since he too, like my patient, falls in love. With much guilt and sadness he realizes that he loves the virginal nun. His fate was decided when he refused to fight in the duel that ended with his death.

In another clinical instance, having an attractive, eye-catching muscular physique became very important to a young man when he broke up with his lover. He enjoyed the admiring and envious glances from other men in the health club where he worked out daily. Getting this kind of attention became as important to him as success in his career. The only thing that exceeded this pleasure was the control and power achieved in taking over another person's lover. The essence of these dynamics, as discovered in the therapy, was a recreation of his being his mother's darling throughout childhood and adolescence. By being the model son, he disappointed neither of his parents. He achieved much scholastic success, and became a very respected academic in a prestigious university. But he always felt weak, small, and inferior. Being admired for his startling physique and his social successes reinstated the sense of inner power and ecstatic specialness he felt with his mother. Power and control in this case were also a means by which he attempted to cope with threatened inner collapse due to the break-up of a relationship with a lover whom he described as "the best person I have ever met." Mourning this loss occupied the first task of that therapy.

Another young man began a behavior pattern in adolescence that consisted of attempting to attract other men in a variety of settings. But when he succeeded, he invariably escaped in a panic. His fantasies at this time consisted of getting even with his abandoning and controlling mother. Now, he was in control and felt very powerful within himself.

DISCUSSION

There are two sorts of data in a study such as this one about Don Juan and Don Juanism, the literary and the clinical. From the standpoint of clinical observations, Fenichel (1945) said analysis of Don Juan types of personality indicated "that their Oedipus Complex is of a particular kind. It is dominated by the pre-genital aim of incorporation, pervaded by narcissistic needs and tinged with sadistic impulses. In other words, the striving for sexual satisfaction is still condensed with the striving for narcissistic supplies in order to maintain self-esteem" (p. 243). In this quotation a predominately oedipal interpretation seems appropriate, but more importantly, it is pointing to a deeper preoedipal configuration. Robbins (1956), Deutsch (1965), and D. McClelland (1975) essentially follow Fenichel's formulations, and his clinical material also emphasizes the narcissistic issues of a man who used women to maintain inner cohesion and prevent collapse of a fragile self. Ethel Person (1986) describes similar behavior in a group of male patients. Pratt (1960) refers to an essentially "infantile need for reunion with the mother" in Don Juanism and the "philandering represents a flight from incest or perhaps from homosexuality" (p. 328). The data in my case, as well as in the homosexual cases, suggest a deeper narcissistic focus. The clinical data are rather sparse in Pratt's paper and the main subject matter is anthropological in nature. Pratt does, however, take into account the punishment of the Trickster as a function of the superego.

The clinical data that are described in this presentation are culled from the transferences observed in psychoanalytic settings and are not literary or anthropological data. Mr. H resembled the legendary Don Juan but did not conform to the dramatic character in that he was potentially capable of love and the capacity to grow, adapt, and develop a lasting relationship. He was able to make use of his positive qualities of personal charm and convert his creative energies from pathological sexual exploits to experiments in parenting, certain home improvement tasks, and animal training. He started the analysis focused on himself and his selfish needs, but he was able to make use of the analysis to renounce this exclusive focus to a significant degree. Control and power issues were paramount in this man's every interaction with others, but especially with those with whom he had made a commitment to become involved. The reason for this behavior was to ensure continuing contact with the idealized mother and restoration of inner cohesion through maintenance of narcissistic supplies. Frustration of his efforts to control me or some more serious interference with the integrity of the transference or other significant relationships led to loss of inner cohesion. He felt helpless to prevent his mother's death. He couldn't prevent his father's angry disappointment in him; his father's advancing age; his father dating; his woman friend dating or her childish neediness, but most importantly separations or empathic failures in the analytic relationship. What usually followed was a temper tantrum that his wishes had to be followed to the letter. The next step was a grandiose fantasy of making large sums of money, but in the process of putting his fantasy into action he engaged in erratic, impulsive self-defeating business practices. Withdrawal, feelings of helplessness, depression, a sleep disorder, lack of energy, and a pervasive sense of fatigue were coupled with a gloomy pessimistic outlook of impending disaster and catastrophe. He felt abandoned and unable to function. On weekends, he rarely set foot out of the house except for brief excursions with his father for breakfast or to his aunt's house for dinner. He felt disconnected from me and struggled to make constructive plans for the future. Years earlier, he had medicated himself with cocaine and marijuana, but now he abused tobacco by smoking large quantities of cigarettes. He was desperate to have a family life, but he was totally unprepared for the compromises and adaptive tasks required of intimate adult relationships in a family. He was more given to trading one thing for another, a kind of bartering: "I'll give you this, if you'll give me that."

In the transference, he felt forced into a helpless submissive–dependent relationship with me that was paralyzing. He thought other patients were more preferred than himself. Control and power were, in fact, used to maintain the continuity of self-cohesion when the threat of regression, fragmentation, or loss of boundaries occurred due to a real or imagined rupture in the primary relationship. My observations, furthermore, led me to think that a massive resistance, clinically manifest as control, occurred in response to a break in the integrity of the wholeness of the self due to separation, or less frequently, failures in empathy in the transference.

What the Don Juan type of character, as clinically observed, strives to preserve at all costs is the internalized image of the idealized mother self–selfobject, which process is acted out with a succession of conquests, none of whom actually can measure up to the idealized mother. The Don Juan behavior began as a sexualization of the repressed affective state that emerged later as an imperfectly obscured depression.

This formulation resembles very closely the one proposed for perversions (Goldberg, 1977, 1995), but Don Juanism does not seem to be a perversion in the usual sense, and more specifically in terms of traditional psychoanalytic theory (Socarides, 1988), except that the unconscious conflicts in the clinical data presented could be characterized as predominately preoedipal in origin. What seems to be cogent is that the Don Juan character presents a kind of *pseudovitality*, a term Kohut used to describe a defensive posture to counteract an "inner deadness and depression. As children, these patients had felt emotionally unresponded to and had tried to overcome their loneliness and depression through erotic and grandiose fantasies" (p. 5). Kohut (1977) referred to the frantic sexual activities of some depressed adolescents as arising under similar circumstances (p. 272). My patient was similar in many respects to this formulation.

On the other hand, the literary Don Juan, like Hamlet, Faust, and Don Quijote are all characters in major works of art (Weinstein, 1967) that continue to present a fertile source of continuing study. Deutsch (1937) characterized Don Quijote also as a narcissistic character, but it must be remembered that the man from *La Mancha* was asexual and was consumed with an idealized world. Mandel's (1963) collection of various versions of the Don Juan play demonstrate that one can observe the changes in the literary Don Juan through the ages and in different cultures that in a way traces the history of Western mankind: "always, he beats with the pulse of his epoch and the reason is that not one literary work concerning him is great enough to have forced a new note on its times or to have deviated into eccentric splendor. The fact must be faced: Don Juan as a type of man remains in the end more interesting than any of the plays, poems, or novels which gave him life" (p. 21). The essential feature of the classical character of Don Juan, according to Mandel (1963), is "supreme sensuality," representing a kind of erotic triumph over other aspects of his character (p. 12). He goes on to specify that this is not just one element in Don Juan's personality, but the essence of his self, "rather it is his life's only business; whatever else he may be or do is incidental" (p. 12). Mandel probably was inspired by Kierkegaard's emphasis on sensuality in Mozart's Don Giovanni and Kierkegaard's own work (1987, pp. 31–113). It has been said that there are as many versions of the legend as there were conquests (according to Lorenzo Da Ponte—"one thousand and three" in Spain alone). Incidentally, one other interesting fact is that Mozart wrote the part for the young adult 22-year-old Luigi Bassi (Moberly, 1967, pp. 196–197).

Similarly, psychoanalytic interpretations have changed over the years with each new theory. Otto Rank (1924) was the first psychoanalyst to make a comprehensive applied psychoanalytic study of the Don Juan legend, using psychoanalytic concepts to bring informed understanding to this curious and fascinating story. He interpreted the story as primarily oedipal, wherein the seduced women represent the unattainable mother and the deceived men as the father. The commander as father metes out retribution as a representation of the superego. Leporello (Catalinon) is seen as the ego ideal. Actually, Catalinon is a comic or jester whose name was known to the audience in sixteenth-century Spain as a feminine one. In the play he is meekly submissive to Don Juan, even though he may warn Don Juan of the dangers of his behavior in ego ideal fashion. Rank's study dealt with the version written by Da Ponte the librettist for Mozart's opera *Don Giovanni*. Parenthetically, it also appears that both Mozart and Da Ponte may have been given to Don Juanlike behavior (Davenport, 1932). It is said, too (Nettl, 1956), that upon Da Ponte's invitation Casanova added a few lines to the libretto (Da Ponte, 1961).

Ferenczi (1922) may have preceded Rank's contribution in his note on "Bridge Symbolism and the Don Juan Legend" which refers to a phallic interpretation. Winter (1973) is intuitively correct about many aspects of his psychological inferences of the Don Juan legend (pp. 168–200), and I agree with him that power and control are important, but there are some notable problems with his formulations as noted above. What is important here is the clinical observation, as in my patient's experience of fusion and a fear of loss of boundaries. In the end, he was comforted by an increasing capacity for closeness and togetherness. Second, Winter's interpretations are derived and inferred from the literary Don Juan and sociopsychological research that is quite important, but is different from clinical data. Finally, Don Juan, like other literary heroes such as Akhilleus or Odysseus, was a figure of action (Don Juan was called the Hector of Seville), but action is not the main characteristic even in the literary character of Don Juan. He is a "spoiled brat" (a *senorito*) who always takes advantage of others and is not capable of taking the sacraments of marriage (Maetzu, 1938). Jose Ortega y Gasset asserts that Don Juan is virility itself and is nothing until he performs sex with a woman. What is so attractive about Don Juan is his "Aladdin of vitality who has the magic lamp of ever conquering energy and the miracle of everlasting power" (Maetzu, 1938, p. 91). As Mandel states,

> The original Don Juan, and the Don Juan of the entire classical period, was a powerful man. He shows this by being so often successful in his tricks, by an extraordinary adeptness with the sword, by (and this is usually overlooked) his wonderful luck,

even by his excellent connections and his noble birth, and by his thrilling defiance of the forces of the supernatural, which the common man is always told to adore but which he does not mind having flouted—by somebody else" [Mandel, 1963, p. 19].

Moberly (1967) quotes Conan Doyle's character Baron Gruner who bragged of a hundred women he seduced. He describes Mozart's Don as:

[A] healthy male animal. He is not just over-sexed. He eats well, drinks well, sees well, has a good sense of smell, is immensely energetic, needs very little sleep. Women respond instinctively to his self-confident presence. He is gay, handsome, wealthy, leisured, well-born, well-dressed, well-mannered; a gentleman in several senses of the word. He has all the advantages, and is a thoroughly irresponsible young fellow. He is therefore out to enjoy a certain ritual. He enjoys it. He ensures that they enjoy it at the time. He is genuinely bewildered that they should be so selfish and narrow-minded as to want to keep him [p. 149].

SUMMARY AND CONCLUSIONS

The opportunity to study certain characteristics in an adult man who began a behavior pattern in adolescence that resembled the legendary and mythical literary character of Don Juan led to this study of a particular form of hypersexuality. It is very interesting that the literary figure of Don Juan has been the subject of many versions of the original plot conceived by Tirso de Molina. This chapter has been devoted to a serious study of the literary character comparing him to clinical material. Power and dominating control issues were signal defenses against a narcissistic depression in this man as seen in his relationships with women and in the transference relationship with me. The transference data have been put to use in providing a formulation for an explanation of the phenomena observed.

Other clinical data concerning women and some homosexual men are presented in a more abbreviated fashion. This research effort is a retrospective construction of the dynamics that led to this man's neurosis.

In my opinion, a self psychological interpretation offers the more felicitous fit than the classical oedipal interpretation alone. In fact, at first I applied interpretations based on classical oedipal theory concerning issues of competition with me as father, and fear of retaliation and castration, but this strategy resulted in little or no response. More important than symptomatic response, however, the data minimally and weakly supported those interpretations. To be sure, there were competitive and phallic oedipal issues. Moreover, when his mother died, he was drawn into a closer relationship with his father and a relationship accompanied by wishes and fantasies of taking his mother's place. These wishes were quite real, but, as the analysis proceeded, this negative oedipal configuration occupied a much less prominent place in the dynamics. Power and control issues dominated the clinical picture masking a depression emanating from a deeper narcissistic focus. Interpretation of these narcissistic issues provided my patient with the relief he was seeking, while the main effect of the sedative medication was to help him to sleep. By giving him something, a deep-seated wish was gratified to get something from me as his father. In a way, frustration of that wish over the years had much to do with cementing the idealized mother transference.

REFERENCES

Austen, J. (1939), *The Story of Don Juan: A Study of the Legend and the Hero.* London: Martin Secker.

Beauvoir, S. de (1985), *Adieux: A Farewell to Sartre,* tr. P. O'Brian. New York: Pantheon.

Danois, Countess (1774), *The Lady's Travels into Spain,* Vol. 1. London: T. Davies.

Da Ponte, L. (1961), *Don Giovanni*, tr. W. H. Auden & C. Kallman. New York: G. Schirmer.

Davenport, M. (1932), *Mozart.* New York: Dorset.

de Molina, T. (1630), Don Juan. In: *Great Spanish Plays in English Translation.* New York: Dover, 1991, pp. 81–133.

Deutsch, H. (1937), Don Quixote and Don Quixotism. *Psychoanal. Quart.,* 6:215–222.

——— (1965), *Neuroses and Character Types.* New York: International Universities Press.

Ellis, H. (1908), *The Soul of Spain.* New York: Houghton Mifflin.

Erikson, E. (1959), Identity and the Life Cycle. *Psychological Issues,* Monogr. 1. New York: International Universities Press.

Fenichel, O. (1945), *The Psychoanalytic Theory of Neuroses.* New York: W. W. Norton.

Ferenczi, S. (1922), Bridge symbolism and the Don Juan legend. In: *Theory and Technique of Psychoanalysis.* New York: Basic Books, 1952, pp. 356–358.

Flores, A. (1991), *Great Spanish Plays in English Translation.* New York: Dover Publications.

Freud, S. (1920), The psychogenesis of a case of homosexuality in a woman. *Standard Edition,* 18:147–172. London: Hogarth Press, 1955.

Goldberg, A. (1975), A fresh look at perverse behavior. *Internat. J. Psycho-Anal.,* 56:335–342.

——— (1995), *Perversion.* Hillside, NJ: Analytic Press.

Horner, A. J. (1989), *The Wish for Power and the Fear of Having It.* Northvale, NJ: Jason Aronson.

Hume, M. (1927), *The Court of Philip IV.* New York: Brentano's.

Kavesh, L., & Lavin, C. (1989), Married, but still wedded to the chase. *Chicago Tribune.* February 1, 5:5.

Kierkegaard, S. (1987), *Either Or,* ed. & tr. H. V. Hong & E. H. Hong. Princeton, NJ: Princeton University Press.

Kohut, H. (1977), *The Restoration of the Self.* New York: International Universities Press.

Kunitz, S. J., & Colby, V. (1967), *European Authors, 1000–1900.* New York: H. W. Wilson.

Laclos, C. de (1782), Les Liaisons Dangereuses. In: *Oeuvres Completes.* Paris: Pleiade.

McClelland, D. C. (1975), *Power and the Inner Experience.* New York: Irvington.

McClelland, I. L. (1967), Don Juan, In: *Encyclopedia Britannica,* Vol. 7. Chicago: Encyclopedia Britannica, p. 586.

Maetzu, R. de (1938), *Don Quijote, Don Juan y la Celestina,* tr. P. A. Brockman & P. J. Cevallos Candau. Madrid: Espasa-Calpe, S. A., Colleccion Austral.

Mandel, O. (1963), *The Theater of Don Juan*. Lincoln: University of Nebraska Press.

Moberly, R. B. (1967), *Three Mozart Operas*. London: Victor Gollancz.

Nettl, P. (1956), Casanova and Don Giovanni. *Saturday Review*, 39:44 and passim. January 28.

Nin, A. (1966–1971), *The Diary of Anais Nin*, Vol. 2, ed. G. Stuhlmann, New York: Swallow.

Person, E. (1986), Male sexuality and power. *Psychoanal. Inqu.*, 6:3–25.

Pratt, D. (1960), The Don Juan Myth. *Amer. Imago.*, 17:321–335.

Rank, O. (1924), *The Don Juan Legend*, tr. & ed. D. G. Winter. Princeton, NJ: Princeton University Press, 1975.

Robbins, L. L. (1956), A contribution to the psychological understanding of the character of Don Juan. *Bull. Menn. Clinic*, 20:166–180.

Shaw, G. B.(1903), *Man and Superman*. New York: Penguin, 1974.

Socarides, C. W. (1988), *The Preoedipal Origin and Psychoanalytic Therapy of Perversions*. Madison, CT: International Universities Press.

Trachtenberg, P. (1988), *The Casanova Complex*. New York: Poseidon.

Weinstein, L. (1967), *The Metamorphosis of Don Juan*. New York: AMS.

Winter, D. G. (1973), *The Power Motive*. New York: Free Press.

Worthington, M. (1962), Don Juan as myth. *J. Lit. & Psychol.*, 12:113–124.

Chapter 6

The Power Motive in Late Adolescence and Young Adulthood

Lord Acton's famous dictum "Power tends to corrupt; absolute power corrupts absolutely" is as true today as on April 5, 1887, when he wrote this phrase in a letter to Bishop Mandell Creighton. Pertinent examples are easily recalled concerning leaders of the greatest of nations throughout history to the smallest of modern institutions.

There are many definitions of *power*,[1,2] but a psychoanalytic definition as it arises in adolescence and young adulthood includes the focusing, channeling, control, and mastery over inner drivenness, helplessness, acquisition of knowledge

---

[1]There are as many definitions of the word *power* as there are different intellectual disciplines: *philosophy* (Hobbes, 1651; Kaufmann, *Encyclopedia Britannica*, 1967; Nietzsche, 1886; Russell, 1969; Mace, 1979; Strauss, 1984; Rawlinson, 1987), *military* (Benson, 1929; Syme, 1939, 1963; Dorey, 1969; Manchester, 1978; Tzu, 1983; Ellis, 1989); *political* (Plutarch, 1909; Robinson, 1916; Dorey, 1969; Strauss, 1984; Smith, 1988); *sociological* (Winter, 1973, 1987; Giddens, 1976; Raven, 1986; Wrong, 1988); and *psychological and psychoanalytic* concepts of power (Freud, 1921; B. Bornstein, 1951; GAP Report, 1978; M. Bornstein, 1986; Grotstein, 1986; Loewenberg, 1986; Olsson, 1986, 1988; Person, 1986; Simon, 1986; Goldberg, 1987; Zimmermann, 1987; Horner, 1989; Klebanow, 1989).

[2]The word *power* in its present spelling came into existence in the fourteenth century (*Oxford Dictionary*) and was derived from the Latin word *potere*, meaning to be able. *Cassell's New Latin Dictionary* (1959, p. 460) derives the word from the Latin *potior* meaning to get possession of, to obtain or to possess and be master of; another Latin origin is *potestas, potestatis,* meaning power to do something, power over something, control as in (1.) supremacy or dominance; (2.) the authority of a magistrate-official authority, office. *Webster's Third New International Dictionary* defines power as being in

(Foucault cited in Rawlinson [1987]) of oneself, the world, and one's creative talents, but also certain capacities for leadership to compel obedience by and dominance over others.

PHILOSOPHY OF POWER

Foucault combined his concept of power with knowledge, saying that power produces knowledge and they imply each other (Rawlinson, 1987). Furthermore, Rawlinson contends that power is fundamentally productive. Nietzsche (1886), like Hobbes (1651) before him, contended that power was a basic drive in all human beings and was *the* essence of the basic human drive. It is the "primitive form of affect, that all other affects are only developments of it" (p. 366). Curiously enough, Nietzsche's idea of will to power seems to be related to Freud's drive theory, but it is not to be confused with Adler's term *will to power* (1956), which he borrowed from Nietzsche but interpreted to be a compensatory structure for organ inferiority or feelings of inferiority that he considered to be a neurotic striving beginning in early infancy and childhood.

Hobbes (1651) concluded in his *Leviathan*³ that there was

> [A] general inclination of all mankind—a perpetual and restless desire of Power after power, that ceaseth only in death and the cause of this, is not always that a man hopes for a more extensive delight, than he has already attained to; or that he cannot be content with a moderate power but because he cannot assure the power and means to live well, which he hath present, without the acquisition of more [pp. 49–50].

Hobbes went on to say that kings assure the continuance of their power at home by laws and abroad by war. For some,

a position of ascendancy; it also implies an ability to compel obedience, control or dominance. It implies physical or mechanical power (horsepower, kilowatts, megatons, or mips-millionth of electronic computer information per second).

³A Leviathan was probably a crocodile or a mythological sea monster that symbolized primeval chaos, mentioned in *The Bible* (Job 3:1; 41:1).

fame is enough and for others "ease and sensual pleasure" . . . [and still others] "admiration and or of being flat-
tered for excellence in some art, or other ability of the mind"
(p. 50). In fact, he traces this drive to one of the cardinal sins,
vanity, that is coupled with ambition and a passion for fame
(Strauss, 1984). In Hobbes's *English Works*, he says "men from
their very birth, and naturally scramble for everything they
covet, and would have all the world, if they could, to fear and
obey them" (Vol. 7, p. 73). The greatest cause of instability in
an institution or organization is a desire for absolute power.
Strauss (1984), a Hobbesian scholar, regarded power as man's
"irrational striving for power, man's natural appetite, [having]
its basis in the pleasure which man takes in the consideration
of his own power, i.e., in vanity" (p. 11) and that power is a
striving for "honor, precedence over others and recognition
of this precedence by others, ambition, pride and the passion
for fame" (p. 11). According to Mace (1979), another Hobbesian scholar, absolute power exists only by consent but at the
same time it is the greatest cause of political instability.

Bertrand Russell's definition of power is that it involves the
production of intended effects (1969), and he is mainly concerned with power over human beings which he divided into
various forms (priestly, naked, and revolutionary). Russell regards the love or desire for power as an "essential part of human nature, and in energetic men it is a very large and
important part" (pp. 262–263); naked power referred to military conquests. For example, McNeill (1984) outlined the use
of naked power throughout history since 1000 A.D. Dennis
Wrong agrees with Russell's definition as "the capacity to produce intended and foreseen effects on others . . ." (1988, p.
21), but he differentiates between power over and power to;
meaning that power over others is different from the capacity
to act on the world. Moreover, Wrong doesn't believe that the
concept of power emanating from either a biological drive or

some universal human psychological characteristic is a very useful or tenable one. For him, power is simply the mobilization by an actor, whether individual or collective, of resources such as wealth, official position, fame, skill, knowledge, etc., to produce desired effects. Wrong is not concerned with power as derived from unconscious motivations, which he regards as just existing.

Giddens (1976) regarded power functionally as a transformative capacity that is tied to action, but is not necessarily coercive. "People are undoubtedly often able to express hostile and aggressive impulses by wielding power over others, but it is usually a highly indirect, canalized and symbolic form of expression. Power is more often sought as a means to other satisfactions such as wealth, sexual gratification, prestige, and a wide range of valued experiences in general" (p. 236).

In modern times, certain ethnic groups have promoted their collective aims, such as African Americans seeking Black Power in the 1960s and 1970s. The energy and the motivation of that social revolutionary movement was largely due to young adult people like the Black Panthers, Martin Luther King, Jr., and Malcolm X. Moreover, some leaders, for example, Jesse Jackson, prepared their young adult sons to assume power in political and governmental organizations. Likewise, King Minos set up his young adult sons in power to bring peace and stability to the region around the Aegean islands and as Thucydides said (quoted by Parry, 1989), "the effect of power and resource is first to create order" (p. 292).

A comprehensive, all-inclusive and exclusive single philosophical definition that covers all pertinent issues would be very cumbersome, but the one Dennis Wrong (1988) proposed, as derived from Bertrand Russell's work (1969), is suitable from a philosophical perspective: "the capacity to produce intended effects on others . . ." (p. 210).

The power of achievement is clearly represented in the adolescent and young adult athlete's activities, where the potential for extraordinary and unforgettable neuromusculoskeletal achievements are practiced to the point of world class competition in various sports (e.g., Jesse Owens, Carl Lewis, Michael Johnson, and Florence Griffith-Joyner in track and Michael Jordan in professional basketball).

POLITICAL POWER

Henry Kissinger is reported to have said that political power is the ultimate aphrodisiac. In our political system, power for Hedrick Smith (1988) means a lot of things.

> In short, the most vital ingredients of power are often the intangibles. Information and knowledge are power. Visibility is power. A sense of timing is power. Trust and integrity are power. Personal energy is power; so is self-confidence. Showmanship is power. Likability is power. Access to the inner sanctum is power. Obstruction and delay are power. Winning is power. Sometimes the illusion of power is power [p. 42].

Reputation is power and having wealth is power. It is interesting to observe in our nation's capital how fluidly the centers of power shift from one individual or group to another, often in a matter of days or hours. Smith (1988) quotes a State Department psychiatrist, Dr. Piecznick, to the effect that many politicians in his experience have a deep sense of loneliness and helplessness that they overcome through their professional activities. It is clear, too, that politicians eagerly crave the spotlight and enjoy being the center of attention. For them rhetoric is power. For example, Hitler's spellbinding marathon oratory at mass meetings excited the German population to a frenzy of emotion that amalgamated them into a powerful national force. Similarly, during the Battle of Britain, Churchill's

speeches inspired the British people to heights of national sac-
rifice and heroism. Bullock (1992) compares the lives of Hitler
and Stalin, both of whom were driven to seek and maintain
absolute power. On the other hand, a much different style was
Franklin Delano Roosevelt's intimate fireside radio talks that
inspired millions of Americans. He was attempting to bypass
power struggles within the administration, with Congress, and
with the judiciary, but Roosevelt's base of power was always
the people, and especially young people, whom he inspired to
overcome the economic depression. Perhaps more so, programs such as the Civil Conservation Corps, Works Progress
Administration, and ultimately the advent of World War II facilitated economic recovery, and in addition it was Roosevelt's
innovative economic policies and his charismatic leadership
that integrated his programs with economic forces that brought
the great depression to a halt.

The written word, though, is powerful in a different way from
the spoken word. For example, Sigmund Freud's work without
doubt influenced Western thought and culture in the twentieth
century, perhaps more than that of any other person. In fact,
Freud himself linked the impact of his discoveries of the unconscious and its motivations on Western thought and culture to
the other major intellectual and scientific discoveries of Darwin
and Copernicus (1917). Alice Kaplan (1995), who has studied
the origins of the French language, asserts that "written language, not speech, is the real site of power. Throughout French
history, the literary function and the political function of writing have been closely tied, and literary figures have made effective critiques of society by reworking and challenging the
writing that came before them" (pp. 48–49). She cites the
enormous outcry and literary outpouring in writings by Zola
and others in the Dreyfus affair of the 1890s.

Winter (1987), who studied the media coverage of presiden-
tial debates, found three different motivations: achievement

(striving for excellence); affiliation-intimacy (concerns about and wishes for close relationships with others); and power-prestige (seeking social power). Using data from projective testing (TAT), he defined power as strong, vigorous actions that have an impact on others, efforts to convince, persuade, offer unsolicited help, and monitor or control; actions that arouse strong reactions in others; and concern for reputation and prestige.

But the person who wrote the bible on power in the sixteenth century was Machiavelli. Scholars from Gentili (1585) to Rousseau (*Social Contract*, 1762) to Donaldson (1988), and quoted by Donaldson, have suggested that Machiavelli was subtly advocating his republican views when he wrote his treatise *Il Principe* (1513a,b), even though he originally wrote it for Guiliano de Medici, the new leader of Florence. But when Guiliano unexpectedly died, Machiavelli dedicated it to Lorenzo de Medici (nephew of Lorenzo the Magnificent) as a manual for heads of state. Machiavelli's first public office was as the second chancellor in the republican government and secretary to the *Ten of War* in Florence. He was then sent as a diplomat to various royal courts throughout Italy and France while he was still a young adult, and thus became intimately acquainted with various behind-the-scenes political and military issues of his time.

It is interesting that Machiavelli advocated the raising of a civilian militia to be kept under civilian control. The soldiers he said should be inculcated with a religious spirit and held to an oath taken on induction. When the republican government was overturned by the Spanish invaders, the Medici were returned to power at the same time Pope Leo X, Giovanni de Medici, was elected to the Holy See, and his brother, Cardinal Giulio de Medici, who later became Pope Clement VI, were all young adults. The two great centers of power of Rome and Florence were then inextricably linked. Machiavelli hoped the new Prince would make it possible to unite these two great cities, and felt it was permissible to use evil means to accomplish this aim.

De Grazia (1989), among others, calls Machiavelli a "staunch republican [but] he is convinced that the times require extraordinary measures taken by one man alone" (p. 240). The Medici family, rich and powerful bankers even before the sixteenth century, used their superior intellectual and financial powers to regain control from the republican majority that had ruled the city for many years. Cosimo, the father of Florence and Lorenzo the Magnificent, and the entire Medici family were known for their maneuvering intrigues and their murderous double-dealing. Machiavelli thought that if anyone could bring the country together a Medici could. Anyone looking today at the imposing statue of Lorenzo in the Uffizi Gallery in Florence cannot fail to be impressed by the strong sense of power and dominance captured in the sculpture. Machiavelli partly sought out the Medicis with *The Prince* (1513a) as a means of ingratiating himself and returning himself to power, but he was never invited back. It is interesting that Machiavelli suggested that military leaders should study history to learn from past successes and failures like Alexander the Great who imitated Akhilleus, Caesar who imitated Alexander, and Scipio who imitated Cyrus (chapter 14, p. 53).

MILITARY POWER

The ancient Chinese military tactician Sun Tzu, probably a group identity (c. 453–221 B.C.), wrote about the strategic essentials of cleverness, boldness, surprise tactics, and intelligent planning for waging war. Alexander the Great, through the vital and energetic leadership that was the source of his power, was the first and youngest military leader to conquer the world as it was known at the time. It is little known, though, that he was the first general to devise a type of medical service for the army and to employ surgeons on the field of battle (Shampo and Kyle, 1982). Four World War II generals come to mind: Montgomery, MacArthur, Patton, and the German general Rommel, the "Desert Fox," of the Afrika Korps (Young, 1960). All four were bold and courageous in battle, thought themselves invincible, invulnerable to danger, and created magnificent myths about themselves. They were unusually creative in combat, using surprise to gain success. General Douglas MacArthur's overinvolved relationship with his ambitious mother was boundaryless. She even moved to a nearby hotel to be near him when he was at West Point and pushed his career at the highest levels in the army wherever and whenever she could (Manchester, 1978). At her insistence, he leaned on her well into adulthood to make the most elementary decisions. For example, all girl friends had to meet her approval before he could date them.

Political leaders, too, create myths and construct mysteries about their administrations that they believe are invincible. These are the *arcana imperii* (a term used by Machiavelli). Syme (1939) described how Augustus Caesar accomplished dominance over the Roman world through military, financial, and political acts. Alcibiades, a military leader in ancient Athens, displayed strong desires for power as a competitive and aggressive adolescent and young adult (Benson, 1929; Plutarch, 1909). He lost both parents at an early age and was taken in by his famous uncle Pericles. He sought and maintained dominance while shifting sides from Athens to Sparta and back again. He was brave in battle and a successful general with both cities. He was also a very handsome Don Juanlike character, publicly flaunting his affairs with both men and women. He married the daughter (Hipparete) of the richest man (Hipponicus) in Athens, and he had a "demonic passion for popularity which he assured himself was certainly not cured. He remained to the end of his life enamored of the limelight, undisciplined and without self-control to choose the worthier cause if the other was the pleasanter, the popular or the more picturesquely devilish" (Benson, 1929, p. 69).

All too often political leaders are corrupt and totally disregard the truth. In fact, Hitler demonstrated that the bigger the lie the more likely it is to be believed. Loewenberg (1986) quotes Fawn Brodie's biography of Nixon that he was "a liar in matters large and small throughout his life. . . . Nixon lied to gain love, to store up his grandiose fantasies, to bolster his ever wavering sense of identity. He lied in attacks, hoping to win . . . and always he lied, and this most aggressively, to deny that he lied . . . finally, he enjoyed lying" (Brodie, 1981, p. 25).

Allen Friedman (Friedman and Schwartz, 1989) described the story of blatant corruption of politicians who were bought off by the powerful Teamsters' Union. He and Schwartz exposed the most seamy aspect of our political system. Lying, stealing, and mayhem were reported to be sanctioned by union officials. Any means were permissible to accomplish their aims.

Klebanow's view of money as power (1989) occurs in her observation of a number of young brokers whose primary interest was to make extraordinary amounts of money, sometimes under less than honest circumstances. Also, some law students in a recent survey stated their sole purpose in entering the legal profession was to make lots of money. In the clinical psychoanalytic setting, Olsson (1986) points out the countertransference difficulties that can arise in analysis with powerful and "phenomenally wealthy" persons. For example, envy and greed are stirred up in the analyst that may lead to further difficulties in the therapy. For the patient, an unconscious regard for money as an entré to immortality, grandiose fantasies, and a sense of entitlement merge with external reality because reality can be readily manipulated with money.

Tacitus described his father-in-law (Agricola), the governor of the Roman province of Britannia: "His appearance was handsome [and] rather imposing; his features showed no forcefulness but very great charm; you would be ready to think he was a good man, and glad to know he was a great one" (Dorey, 1986, p. 2). Tacitus went on to describe Agricola as having been steeped in philosophy and possessing moderation and practical wisdom, qualities that are "indispensable to statesmanship" (Dorey, 1986, p. 10). Humanity and merci-fulness complemented Agricola's other qualifications as gov-ernor.

In fact, most political leaders are driven not always by selfish motives but by the desire to deliver a better life to the people they represent. Kohut in his paper "On Leadership" (1985) described the unconscious fantasies of the group that merges with the leader's grandiose fantasies of greatness and power, a concept different from the classical view of identifying with the leader's ideals.

In contrast to these and many other altruistic leaders, a pathological distortion of altruistic ideals has been represented in those cultist leaders like Charles Manson, David Koresh, and Jim Jones. Olsson (1988) described similar dynamics of the terrorist from a developmental point of view. He quotes Cor-rado's (1981) idea that the terrorist "exclusively and explicitly [uses] political tactic[s] employed by self-appointed individuals who operate in small clandestine groups and want to overthrow existing societal institutions through economic, social, and po-litical chaos" (Olsson, 1988, p. 294). The terrorist's grandiose nuclear self merges with an extended national identity, flag, religious organizations, and ethnicity which when injured can "feed the pathological forms of a grandiose self via embla-zoned images of revenge, reverberating, destructive power in dramatized terror" (Olsson, 1988, p. 52). The media are often skillfully used for shock value to promote the strategic aims of the "self-appointed martyr, savior, or messiah. The terrorist feels himself or herself to be the personification of ethnic or nationalistic expression of a group's fantasied liberation or historical destiny" (Olsson, 1988, p. 54).

Loewenberg (1986) examined the careers of Nixon and Hitler from the standpoint of libido theory and ego psychology. He pointed out the many ego strengths in both men which contributed to their attaining great power, but they both succumbed to even stronger self-defeating tendencies, which Loewenberg attributes to guilt about success. What is clear from Loewenberg's account of these men's lives, however, is that both men had very close relationships with their mothers. It is to be remembered that Nixon referred to his mother as a saint. Loewenberg (p. 33) quotes Waite's (1977) work on Hitler that documents an early "incestuous relationship" with his overindulging mother, exposure to the primal scene, and possible rape of the mother by the brutal father. Hitler wore a picture of his mother on his chest (Hamilton, 1978). In addition, the story has been reported that Hitler's mother was badly treated by a Jewish doctor with iodoform gauze instead of surgery for cancer of the breast. Her alleged premature iatrogenic death (when he was 18) has been blamed as the apparent basis for Hitler's anti-Semitism. Loewenberg refers to Erikson's hypothesis that Hitler created a myth of an immortal adolescent who never gave in to adversity and that of an older protective and celibate brother—Der Führer, the leader. Loewenberg said this was "a major feat of synthesis, creativity and adaptation" (p. 38). He used his fantasy life to construct a political movement mixed with a folk style religion based on the invincible nature of a pure race. He used ritualized mass meetings, his love for the mysticism of Wagnerian opera, and a kind of holy war with the enemy, being the Jews. Hitler, it is well known now, suffered from hypochondriacal delusions that he had cancer of the stomach, and had fears of an inner collapse which finally he succumbed to with his suicide. Of course, not all political leaders have this kind of psychopathology, but a closer examination of the strivings for power in political leaders is begging for explication.

So much for philosophical, political, and military power. But so far we are lacking a suitable integration of the concept of power in the mainstream of psychoanalytic theory. Bringing some modest change in that situation is the goal of this chapter. The thesis here about power is similar to the dynamics delineated in the Don Juan chapter. But the big difference here is that power is not sexualized as in the Don Juan character. What makes one individual mad for power and another seek sexual dominance is very complex, but it seems one major dynamic is that the latter were most likely overstimulated in childhood by an intensely sexualized relationship with their mothers, while those who seek nonsexualized dominance were intensely involved with their mothers as grandiose self-selfobjects in struggles for power and control. They had engaged in a basic merger with the omnipotent and omniscient mother selfobject when the infant and child were helpless and totally dependent on her for survival. Later on, both types of individuals were disappointed and disillusioned with their fathers as a resource to assist in an escape from the mother–child dyad, whether mother was seductive or controlling. Moreover, the fathers of both types failed to assist their children in negotiating the developmental tasks of childhood and adolescence on into young adulthood, being particularly pathogenic in dealing with oedipal issues in childhood and adolescence. This places the issues concerned squarely in the middle of the first *and* second separation–individuation developmental phases (Mahler, 1965, 1968; Mahler, Pine, and Bergman, 1975; Blos, 1979; Isay, 1980; Brockman, 1984; see also chapter 1), the phallic–narcissistic, and oedipal phases of development. Both McClelland (1975) and Deutsch (1967) point to the child's perception of the mother as the giver of strength and resources in the prephallic phase. The following are condensed vignettes selected from more than thirty years of clinical practice where power issues are manifest.

CLINICAL DATA

Mr. G, a 19-year-old adolescent, was hospitalized for drug abuse in the early 1950s. He was a jazz musician, and a minor contributor to the avant-garde of popular music makers of that era. When we began our psychotherapeutic work, he was very resistant because he experienced me as a controlling authoritarian representative of his parents. In a way, he was correct because I had inadvertently chosen to take a stand against his drug abuse. What I didn't realize at the time of hospitalization was that his use of drugs was an attempt to counteract his parents' intrusiveness and their desire to control his career choice, and indeed every aspect of his life. They wanted him to enter one of the professions like any normal Jewish boy and marry within the faith. In the main, intrusiveness was instigated by the mother more so than the father. She laid out his clothes every day and went through his dresser regularly, neatly rearranging the contents while searching for drugs. Her true motive, instead, seemed to express her unwillingness to relinquish her controlling self–selfobject relationship with her son that began in early infancy. He dealt with his parents' intrusiveness by withdrawing and lying about the identity of his friends and his drug use, but this strategy failed to prevent his parents' intrusiveness. When this boundaryless, ambivalent relationship with his mother was addressed in the psychotherapy, and as the crucial rupture in the transference with me was repaired, he learned to trust me and began a longer process of weaning himself away from drugs and his parents.

His use of heroin seemed to recreate the fantasized and perceived bliss of an early infantile merger with his omnipotent and omniscient mother. As the therapy took hold, he picked up the struggle to separate from her. He was significantly able to achieve more autonomy and control over his own life as the neurotic adolescent self gave way to the therapeutically facilitated consolidation of a healthier, integrated young adult personality. He changed his career choice when he realized his musical talents were quite adequate but not at all exceptional. Moreover, he understood that he could not support himself on his musical talents. He was then able to retain his interest in modern music as an avocation. Finally, he became involved in a satisfyingly intimate relationship with an appropriate young woman.

A successful politician, Mr. C was born into a political family dynasty. The father, grandfather, and assorted other relatives had been actively prominent in a dominant statewide political group. His presenting symptoms were severe bouts of depression with suicidal thoughts, anxiety attacks, insomnia, and addiction to drugs and alcohol. These symptoms were complicated by a severely ambivalent and conflicted marriage that involved multiple separations. As the analysis explored repressed, unconscious issues, we discovered that he had been severely traumatized in latency by his parents' violent arguments and subsequent divorce. After the divorce, he remained with his mother and older sister. The mother compensated by being overly indulgent with him from latency on into late adolescence. When he was drafted into the army, he discovered his fiancée was pregnant. Both were unprepared for parenthood and adulthood. Later on, his mother continued to indulge him by buying him expensive clothes and jewelry. In an attempt to recreate and maintain this merger with the indulgent mother, he continued to be self-indulgent by purchasing expensive jewelry, shoes, elaborate belt buckles, and sunglasses. Interestingly, he was an avid student of the lives of powerful political men and charismatic musicians. Analysis of his rich dream life revealed his pursuit of power in government to replace the bountiful mother who relieved his every need. Alcohol and drugs also served immediate gratification of unconscious tension states that were experienced as urgent demands similar to the child's needs for tension reduction.

Mr. F began an analysis in the midst of a major crisis. His marriage was falling apart and job loss was imminent. He felt helpless and unable to control anything in his life. He couldn't calm himself down. He felt powerless. He turned to pornographic movies to relieve the tensions generated by the collapse of the external world as he knew it, combined with the collapse of his internal world too. When he rightly or wrongly perceived empathic failures in the transference situation, he experienced the same panic. Beginning in adolescence, he drew pictures of nude women to stimulate himself. Later on, he went to pornographic movies and bought pornographic magazines. He was loaded down with unbearable shame and guilt after each failure to control his impulses. Before analysis he had no other way to relieve inner tension. When he finally lost his job and was literally kicked out of his house, he went into a massive panic. He felt he had no one on his side since his wife had succeeded in alienating his two teenage children from him. He had no friends. He was severely depressed and felt himself powerless to control anything in his life and especially his regressive symptoms of withdrawal, masturbatory fantasies, hypochondriacal fears, overeating, and compulsive memorizing of poetry and lengthy passages from Shakespeare's plays.

We constructed a childhood where he experienced his mother as emotionally cold and his father as humiliating and competitive with him as a real rival. He grew up seeing his mother's nude body as she went to and from the bath. He experienced these sexually stimulating scenes as warm feelings of pseudocloseness. It is this vision of the mother's nude body that he attempted to recreate in the fantasized omnipotent relationship with the mother through the pornographic movie and masturbatory sexual behavior. As she did the family laundry, he recalled clinging to her legs, attempting to extract what little comfort and closeness he could get.

He was unable to control his excessive drinking as a young adult. Psychotherapy with a dynamically oriented psychiatrist assisted him to regain control over that symptom. Earlier, as an adolescent, he was so shy he was afraid to approach girls and admired them but from a distance. He succeeded in gaining some measure of personality strength and sense of power over his impulses and some part of external reality when he excelled in his father's sport, epitomized when he defeated the state tennis champion. Selectively, intellectual skills were delayed in developing as well as underutilized until graduate school where he was at the top of his class at a prestigious Eastern business school.

Analysis has delivered a healthier self-regard by enabling him to gain enough self-control, insight, and power over his perversion so that the regressive symptoms have all but disappeared and have been replaced with a more normal sex life. He has entered a business that has proved to be very successful.

As a college student, H returned home every weekend to renew and restore his perception of himself as a lovable and admirable whole person. During the week, he felt his grip on this perception of himself slipping away. Though he was not a recluse, his relationships with people at school were sparse and constricted. He would respond appropriately when approached, but he felt ill-equipped to use his considerable intellectual and personal charm. He felt powerless to change anything in his life. He started a second analysis in adulthood because of the persistence of a bothersome passivity, loneliness, depression, and powerlessness to change. Severe insomnia aggravated his depressive affective state. Psychoanalytic investigation of his unconscious motivations revealed the morbidly embarrassing fact that as a latency age boy when he was separated from his parents and sent to live with a grandparent, he was forced into what he perceived and experienced to be a humiliatingly submissive relationship and he was deathly afraid his schoolmates would discover what he had to keep secret. When he moved back with his parents as a preadolescent boy some of the earlier damage was repaired or in the very least covered over. The first analysis had been a helpful, but insufficient working through of the underlying shame and blunting of his aggressive, assertive, masculine identity. Feelings of powerlessness and painful passive submissiveness to all women were traced to the overwhelmingly powerful maternal image that was manifested as low self-esteem and a weakened self-image. The pervasive sense of shame gradually gave way to the analytic process that strengthened and solidified a cohesive masculine assertive self so that his considerable intellectual and personality skills were restored, along with an enduring healthy sense of self-regard.

DISCUSSION

First of all, motivation for power involves many developmental issues. Second, the revival or continuation of earlier developmental conflicts occur during adolescence (Brockman, 1984; see also chapter 1, 5). Competition and oedipal rivalry stimulate guilt and retaliation (castration) anxiety. Shame about failures to achieve one's goals or meeting one's ideals are most common. Moreover, it must be remembered that adolescence is considered to be a second separation–individuation phase of development (Blos, 1979; Isay, 1980). Third, important multiple considerations and integrations of ego and superego development cannot be ignored, but this study is limited to those pertinent and significant issues that have been neglected and underappreciated in previous studies of the consolidation of *power* motivations during adolescence and young adulthood.

Another reason for the study of power motivations is that in modern Western societies, individuals and corporations wield great power over their employees through threats of termination, withholding or dispensing salary increases and bonuses. Furthermore, women in the work force are seriously affected by this state of affairs. Money is power: many women are inhibited and literally prevented from realizing their potential in their business careers or demanding their just due in divorce settlements (Klebanow, 1989). Kestenbaum's (1986) clinical observations of the neurotic dilemma some women have can only be resolved by analysis with a woman analyst to develop the appropriate kind of transferences that can be interpreted while the female analyst can serve as a real role model.

In terms of group psychology (GAP Report, 1978), power is "defined as the capacity to make individuals or groups do what they would rather not do by exerting force or the threat of force, to impose a decision unilaterally" (p. 62). But the validity of power depends on the moral rightfulness of a leader whose authority is supported by a common ideal and a belief system of the people—an idea originally proposed by Freud in *Group Psychology and the Analysis of the Ego* (1921). Freud indicated the power of the leader is related to his exacting obeisance from the members of the primal family by demanding exclusive sexual rights over the available females.

In discussing the founding and growth of a psychoanalytic institute, David Zimmermann (1987) likened power needs to needs for prestige, and compared these processes to the institution of marriage and family life wherein members of the family group attempt to influence others in the family to accomplish individual aims. Occasionally, some members of a psychoanalytic group are more motivated for prestige and power than others. As a matter of fact, power is sometimes sought after more than economic goals, but in the exceptional case money and power over others are combined. Moreover, power cliques tend to form around transference–countertransference connections between training analysts who proselytize their analysands and supervisees. Also, the danger of a structure becoming rigidly fixed on ideological positions reflects the group's anxiety, and insecurity, and the unconscious need of the members to defend themselves against powerlessness, infantile helplessness, and the uncertainty of not knowing everything. In contrast, a healthy structure tolerates theoretical differences and promotes free dialogue within the group as well as reaching out to others outside the group to establish communications with a wider audience.

Interest in the power motive was represented in a group of papers by David Winter (1973, 1987), D. C. McClelland (1975) and the already mentioned GAP report (1978). Winter's and McClelland's data were based on projective tests (TAT and Draw-a-Picture) and questionnaires of a volunteer population of presumptively normal or nonclinical adolescents and young adults. McClelland's definition is a simple feeling of having power. McClelland (1975) traced the inner experience of power to a prephallic stage in which the mother is perceived as the giver of strength and resources, a point of view similar to the thesis derived from clinical data in this paper. Grotstein (1986) described the parameters of powerlessness in terms of deficit or deficiency disorders or in terms of the vicissitudes of drives versus ego defenses. Horner (1996) calls the power motive a wish to overcome infantile helplessness. Adolescents attempt to undo infantile dependence and helplessness by compensatory efforts at mastery to achieve power.

A special issue of *Psychoanalytic Inquiry* (M. Bornstein, 1986) was devoted to power and the editor's conclusion was that traditional instinctual theories "of aggression and sadism, or anxiety and defense are inadequate to deal with the causality and phenomenology of power" (p. 133). Bornstein (1986) believes a psychoanalytic study of power must include a thorough consideration of ego functions, interpersonal relations, and sexual identity. In fact, Ethel Person (1986) emphasizes narcissistic and adolescent developmental issues in her work with four male patients whose macho behavior was characterized by much concern over helplessness and acting out of power issues. Historically, however, psychoanalytic definitions of power as a human motivation have included concepts of a driving force to explore, for mastery, for control over the environment and other persons and for some, an all consuming striving for fame. In fact, Freud (1920, 1921, 1930) considered power to be part of and a derivative of the aggressive drive and ultimately the controversial concept of a death instinct. Ives Hendrick's (1942) concept of the ego instinct of mastery is related to Freud's ego-instincts for self-preservation and survival. In the first two years of life, Hendrick asserts that the instinct to master is an inborn drive to learn how to do various tasks. Dorey (1986) based his concept of power on Freud's instinct theory in terms of mastery-domination versus mastery-assimilation: mastery-domination or *bemachtigungstreib* (Springer, 1974) meaning seizure, to take possession of, and mastery (Freud, 1924), and mastery-assimilation or *bewaltigung* (Springer, 1974) meaning internal mastery of overwhelming tension (Freud, 1920). This metapsychological pair is somewhat confusing and the death instinct theory is somewhat discredited. In fact, Kohut (1977) considered aggression to be primarily secondary to frustration of the child's "demands for total control over the self-object's responses; it demands perfect empathy" (p. 91). Dell (1989), too, follows the Kohutian concept that power is not fundamental but rather is "a highly visible epiphenomenon or some other, perhaps more basic process" (p. 10) and links it to empathic failures in the parents. Kohut (1985, p. 56) speculated about the psychology of group leaders such as in Nazi Germany: "Certain charismatic leaders appear to have been exposed to narcissistic deprivations in early childhood that prevented the gradual modification of their grandiose self and its integration with the reality ego, thus depriving this structure of one of its most important constituents. The leader then:

> Develops a heightened sensitivity to the anonymous group and its motivations and is able to relate to it intensely . . . [when the] fantasies, wishes, and fears of the group . . . are like his own. The unconscious fantasies of the group's grandiose self, expressed in the transference upon the image of an appropriate leader figure, thus can play at times a crucial role in its cohesion. The leader of such a group is not primarily the focal point of shared values, as Freud suggested, but self-righteously expresses the group's ambitions and extols its greatness and power. Along with the various political, social, and economic factors that account for the irresistible attractions which nationalistic movements are able to exert at certain historical junctures, there is thus a psychological one. At certain historical moments there exists a widespread, painful awareness of narcissistic imbalance in large segments of a country's population. Shame propensity and readiness for rage are ubiquitous. Individuals seek to melt into the body of a powerful nation (as symbolized by a grandiose leader) to cure their shame and provide them with a feeling of enormous strength, to which they react with relief and triumph. Old fantasies of omnipotence seem suddenly to have become a reality; all are proclaiming the invincible strength of a nation, and he who dares to question the omnipotence of the group and the omniscience of its leader is an outcast, an enemy, a traitor [p. 57].

DEVELOPMENTAL CONSIDERATIONS

Increasingly, psychoanalysts have turned to the developmentalists for answers to these confusing and contradictory concepts arising in adults undergoing analysis. In order to remain conversant with other disciplines, psychoanalysis should remain open to new findings from infant and child observations as well as new findings in neuroscience, and not be contradictory to these two fields of inquiry (Pine, 1985). As a matter of fact, the developmental point of view offers a rich menu from which to study the origins of the power motive. Beginning in the period of infantile helplessness, what is observed is rage precipitated by separations and frustrations of desires. Squirming to move away from the enclosing embrace of a caretaker and refusal of food could be considered as anlagen for efforts at autonomy and the gaining of power, besides the child's more obvious strivings reflexively or otherwise to exercise his or her back muscles. Conflicts arising from this period occur when the caretaker's need for nurturance is greater than that of the infant and is perpetuated through forced compliance. A child growing up in this family situation becomes excessively alert to behavioral cues and unconscious communications to meet the caretaker's needs, and in adolescence and adulthood feels cheated and deprived.

Proceeding through the toilet-training period there is a variety of behaviors such as anal retentiveness, encopresis, enuresis, and issues of territoriality. Self boundaries are being established and ownership of possessions is jealously guarded, while at the same time the young child is invading others' boundaries and taking their possessions. The struggles for power between mother and child in the anal period are legendary. If the parents, for example, have unfinished narcissistic issues of feeling their children burdensome, and prematurely force them into too independent functioning, then when these children reach adolescence and adulthood there is much rage and acrimony against the parents. A variety of regressive behaviors can be the result, such as aggressive and violent behavior, passive–aggressive behavior, sullenness, or withdrawal to magical thought as a means to exert power over reality.

In the phallic period, urethral exhibitionistic (height and length of urinary stream), and penile competitiveness (little boys humiliating little girls by claiming superiority through possession of a penis) are classical examples of the power motive in operation. In latency, between 8 and 10 years, an extraordinarily important event takes place in terms of the disillusionment of the omnipotence of adults (B. Bornstein, 1951, p. 281). This disillusionment adds to the infantile terror of loneliness, abandonment, helplessness, and powerlessness.

In adolescence, both boys and girls try their strength and test their parents' control, patience, and power. The 1978 GAP report reviews these developmental issues in some detail, and a very creative section on negotiation graphically describes how the struggles for power and dominance in the family can be successfully met and worked through. Incidentally, what is advocated there can be of immense help to therapists confronted with this problem in disturbed, hospitalized adolescents where negotiation and behavioral modification techniques are part of the therapeutic milieu, and in adult analysis as well (Goldberg, 1987). The six useful applications of the negotiation model for parents with adolescents and young adults as discussed in the GAP report are:

1. Empirical testing out of negotiation "to discover confusions and contradictions in the parents' use of authority, especially in disorganized homes" (pp. 243–244). It also helps parents to realize the "goals and objectives of control, limit-setting, discipline, and punishment." Parents and adolescents can question and disagree.
2. "Direct exchange to resolve disagreement and bargaining to remove obstacles and achieve progress" (p. 245). For example, working together to earn freedoms versus overturning authority by rebellion or abdication of authority by the parents or other authority.

3. Establishing a relative parity that is equivalent but not identical with mutual respect "prevents over or undervaluing one another" (pp. 245–246). This is a team approach that prevents blaming or undermining each other.
4. Focusing on the current conflicts brings them out in the open, such as drug use, sex, political activities, issues of racism, work ethics, and middle-class values.
5. Negotiation promotes a "structured and controlled technique to resolve ambivalences and the parties strive to reach reasonable goals" (p. 247) with angry and aggressive conflicts and can stimulate forgiveness on both sides.
6. Negotiation counteracts you versus me and converts it to us, we, our, and identifying with each other's goals to produce mutuality, and helps adolescents and young adults to gain access to and learn how to make decisions, and use power and authority.

These negotiation techniques also apply to residential schools, correctional homes, and therapeutic institutions.

Lichtenberg (1989) outlined what he considered to be the major motivational systems early in development. First, is the attachment–affiliation system, parts I and II, that describes the infant and 1-year-old's development of a psychological and social set of interactive patterns. In part I of the attachment–affiliation system, the newborn infant begins a process of responding to and interacting with the significant caretaker. Lichtenberg assumes with Stern (1977) that there is a nascent separate self that develops a greater sense of separateness and volition as the parental pair gain in confidence with each other to soothe and protect the helpless infant from harm, hunger, and under- or overstimulation. What facilitates the development of attachment and affiliation are the myriad of communications that transpire between mother and infant. Affects and evidence of memory, even in 8-day-old infants, appear to be strong enough indication of a developing agency of the self as an infant becomes attached to its mother.

Part II of the attachment–affiliation phase begins around one year. Failures in tension regulation from this period occur when the caretaker's need for nurturance is greater than that of the infant and is perpetuated through forced compliance. A child growing up in this situation becomes excessively alert to behavioral cues and unconscious communications to preeminently meet the mother's needs, but then in adolescence and young adulthood he feels cheated and deprived of the sustaining growth-producing, modulated interactions between mother and infant. The explorative–assertive system that includes competence and mastery, corresponds to and seems similar (though Lichtenberg would not agree) to the motivation for power as derived from the Freudian aggressive drive. Next is the exploratory–assertive phase that is followed by the aversive–motivational system and the sensual–sexual motivational system.

Emde's (1983, 1988) observations of the earliest motivations in infancy and childhood led him to consider various inborn biologically preadaptive tendencies to be basic motivations: activity, self-regulation, social fittedness, and affect monitoring. More complex early evidence of moral motivations concerning do's and don't's, rule making and turn taking, involve the emotions of joy, fear, anger, sadness, and disgust. However, these early basic motivations undergo multiple modifications throughout childhood and adolescence, and the connection of these observations to late adolescence and young adulthood is very suggestive that infantile exploratory activities, anal, verbal, and moral motivations appear around the same time. The mutual approach and withdrawal dance between mother and infant occurring around 6 months is inextricably connected to the infant's efforts to optimally regulate the incoming stimulation of social interactions that lead to biologically built-in schemas that are "mutually effective in initiating, manipulating, terminating, and avoiding interactions with his mother. He has learned different discursive or dialogue modes, such as turn taking" (Stern, 1977, p. 6). Affective attunement (Stern, 1985, p. 140) can be understood to be another important ingredient in the repertoire of the infant's interactions with his or her caregivers that later may form the basis for power manipulations.

Considered from a developmental point of view, then, the power motive in adolescence and young adulthood is a fertile focus for studying one of the most important nodal points on the path to full adulthood. The acquisition and practicing of those special interpersonal skills that ultimately lead to dominance over others and psychological power, take shape and consolidate in the adolescent period as the culmination of a multitude of earlier developmental achievements. The clinical observations, described synoptically in the previous section of this paper, lead to the conclusion that pathological distortions of power issues in the main arise from a set of dynamics that resemble and remind one of a prephallic attempt to unite with an omnipotent maternal object to relieve the childhood terror of powerlessness, fears of abandonment, and helplessness. This search for a union is further solidified when the father was unavailable to assist the son in separating from the dominating, controlling mother as a preoedipal and oedipal object. The child is then unlikely to internalize those identifications with a strong father that are so necessary for a fuller masculine identity formation and a stronger cohesive self.

This study of the power motive grew out of an interest in the Don Juan character (see chapter 5). More specifically, the Don Juan character achieves power over women as he searches for and merges with the omnipotent idealized mother. Helpless and frightened, experiences of childhood are sexualized. That same motive for merging with the omnipotent mother plays a significant role in seeking power in nonsexualized areas of personality functioning too. This is the significant factor in the psychological life of certain persons seeking political power in government, academic institutions, or other organizations. Political power in national and international circles is especially attractive to some.

The dominant transference pattern of dynamics in those pathological clinical instances of strivings for power cited above, and others that I have encountered in over thirty years of psychoanalytic practice, is indeed that of unconsciously seeking to merge with the internal image of the omnipotent mother. In infancy, she is perceived to be the source of omnipotence and the giver of strength and resources (McClelland, 1975; Deutsch, 1967). It is she who controls the child's every move from morning to night and sometimes throughout the night. No one else can bring the same kind of soothing comfort and sustenance when the child is anxious or hungry. Clinical observations support the assertion that these same issues persist throughout development into adulthood in some persons, albeit in some modified form. These issues were repeated in the regressive analytic situation when separations and loss as well as empathic failures in the transference (real or perceived) produced withdrawal and various regressive forms of psychopathology. Perverse behavior, substance abuse, passivity, obsessive heterosexual or homosexual fantasies and fears, paranoid thinking, hypochondriasis, and rage attacks are some of the resulting symptoms that were observed. For example, perversity, hypochondriasis, insomnia, and drug use were reported to be part of Hitler's psychopathology.

In the clinical psychoanalytic situation, the analyst is perceived to possess an enormous degree of power over his analysand during the regressive phases of the psychoanalytic process in terms of his greater knowledge and insight. He is perceived to control the outcome and know what the analysand must do to be well. Ideally, it is the aim of the analyst to facilitate the transformation of internal conflicts about pathological strivings for power, dominance, and control over others into constructive uses of power, insight, self-knowledge, and identity formation. This achievement might also be considered another form of the transformation of pathological narcissism (Kohut, 1966) into healthy self-realization of latent native talents and conflict energies for exploration, feelings of competence with motor skills, and cognitive capacities (Pine, 1985).

Raven (1986, 1993) developed, along with J. R. P. French (1956), six bases for power in the clinical situation: coercion, reward, legitimacy, expertise, reference, and information. These bases apply equally well to husband/wife, teacher/student, male/female, citizen/bureaucrat, child/playmate, nurse/doctor, and doctor/patient. Power issues arising in intimate relationships between the sexes when studied sociologically yield similar results with some interesting additions (Howard, Blumstein, and Schwartz, 1986). Howard et al. found six dimensions of influence tactics: manipulation, supplication, bullying, autocracy, disengagement, and bargaining, each dimension possessing some more specific variations.

POWER IN ART

Michelangelo's famous statues of Moses and David convey similar perceptions of power. Moreover, his monumental fresco paintings on the Sistine Chapel ceiling constitute an overwhelmingly powerful and impressive piece of work (Oremland, 1989). Art, in fact, can be used to make powerful political statements, especially when Picasso's monumental *Guernica* or the prodigious work of Goya depicting the horrors of the previous civil war in Spain are considered. Even more striking are the great portraitists such as Leonardo, Rembrandt, Franz Hals, and Holbein, who have captured the essence of the personalities of their subjects. Freud's study of both Michelangelo's *Moses* and Leonardo points to the flawed, powerless relationship with their mothers and their attempt to regain that power through their art.

SUMMARY AND CONCLUSIONS

From the clinical data, one pathological dynamic feature stands out among other considerations. What is so prevalent is a reunion or merger with a fantasized omnipotent internal imago of the mother. In the clinical situation this occurs most frequently when there is a threatened or actual disequilibrium in the patient's personality that leads to symptoms associated with feelings of abandonment, loneliness, helplessness, and powerlessness. This condition can be reproduced clinically by separations or empathic failures in the transference–countertransference situation. The presence of a reasonably continuous source of narcissistic supplies from the analyst's comprehensive and resonating understanding resembles the original, but now an internalized omnipotent mother that is therapeutically necessary to maintain and sustain an internal self-cohesion and an inner sense of power and control. Substance abuse, perverse sexual behavior, passivity, sexual fantasies, homosexual fears, paranoid thinking, hypochondriasis, and rage attacks are some of the range of symptomatology experienced during separations and when the analyst fails to appreciate and interpret the psychodynamics of the transference.

I have focused here on the late adolescent and young adult phase of development to study the power motive, because power issues are beginning to consolidate most commonly at this time as derived from earlier developmental antecedents. Fuller consolidation of those capacities for power is completed in young adulthood and adulthood. Ego, ego ideal, and superego structures contribute to this developmental achievement too.

Finally, there are almost always altruistic motives present in political leaders who have a remarkably uncanny and intuitive awareness of what their constituents want at any particular time. They are then often able to match up their goals with the wishes of the majority and give expression to whatever degrees of altruism they possess at any given time. The leader also matches up with the followers' grandiose fantasies or needs for an idealized other.

This set of dynamics is similar to the one suggested for the Don Juan character (chapter 5), except there power is sexualized. Lying to achieve his sexual domination was a feature similar to the nonsexualized behavior of some military and political leaders. A mythic and mysterious story about themselves—the *arcana imperii* of Machiavelli—is created, and military leaders such as the American Army generals MacArthur and Patton and the German general Rommel promoted their mythic invincibility. What differentiates the individual who craves political power is an internal representation built up of experiences that promote power and control over others, but is not sexualized.

REFERENCES

Amplified Old Testament (1962), Grand Rapids, MI: Sonderban.

Adler, A. (1956), *The Individual Psychology of Alfred Adler*, ed. H. L. Ansbacher & R. R. Ansbacher. New York: Basic Books, 1980.

Benson, E. F. (1929), *The Life of Alcibiades*. London: Ernst Benn.

Bornstein, B. (1951), On latency. *The Psychoanalytic Study of the Child*, 6:279–285. New York: International Universities Press.

Bornstein, M. (1986), An epilogue. *Psychoanal. Inqu.*, 6:133.

Blos, P. (1979), *Adolescent Passage*. New York: International Universities Press.

Brockman, D. D., Ed. (1984), *Late Adolescence: Psychoanalytic Studies*. New York: International Universities Press.

Brodie, F. M. (1981), *Richard Nixon: The Shaping of His Character*. New York: W. W. Norton.

Bullock, A. (1992), *Parallel Lives*. New York: Knopf.

Corrado, R. R.(1981), A critique of the mental disorder perspective of political terrorism. *Internat. J. Law & Psych.*, 4:293–308.

De Grazia, S. (1989), *Machiavelli in Hell.* Princeton, NJ: Princeton University Press.

Dell, P. F. (1989), Violence and the systemic view: The problem of power. *Fam. Process*, 28:1–14.

Deutsch, H. (1967), *Selected Problems of Adolescence.* New York: International Universities Press.

Donaldson, P. S. (1988), The relationship of mastery. *Internat. Rev. Psychoanal.*, 13:323–332.

Dorey, R. (1986), The relationship of mastery. *Internat. Rev. Psychoanal.*, 13:323–332.

Ellis, W. M (1989), *Alcibiades.* New York: Routledge.

Emde, R. N. (1983), The prerepresentational self and its affective core. *The Psychoanalytic Study of the Child.* 38:165–192. New Haven, CT: Yale University Press.

—— (1988), Development terminable and interminable. I. Innate and motivational factors from infancy. *Internat. J. Psycho-Anal.*, 69:23–42.

Encyclopedia Britannica, c.v. Kaufmann, W., "Friedrich Nietzsche."

French, J. R. P. (1956), A formal theory of social power. *Psychol. Rev.*, 63:181–194.

Freud, S. (1917), A difficulty in the path of psychoanalysis. *Standard Edition*, 17:135–144. London: Hogarth Press, 1955.

—— (1920), Beyond the Pleasure Principle. *Standard Edition*, 18:3–64. London: Hogarth Press, 1955.

—— (1921), Group Psychology and the Analysis of the Ego. *Standard Edition*, 18:65–143. London: Hogarth Press, 1955.

—— (1924), The economic problem of masochism. *Standard Edition*, 19:155–170. London: Hogarth Press, 1961.

—— (1930), Civilization and Its Discontents. *Standard Edition*, 21:57–145. London: Hogarth Press, 1961.

Friedman, A., & Schwartz, T. (1989), *Power and Greed.* New York: Franklin Watts.

GAP Report 101 (1978), *Power and Authority in Adolescence: The Origins and Intergenerational Conflict*, 10:61–273. New York: Group for Advancement of Psychiatry.

Gentili, A. (1585), *Civil Law, Roman Law, Diplomatic Privileges, and Immunities.* London: Excudebat Thomas Vautrollerius.

Giddens, A. (1976), *New Rules of Sociological Method.* New York: Basic Books.

Goldberg, A. (1987), Psychoanalysis and negotiation. *Psychoanal. Quart.*, 56:109–129.

Grotstein, J. S. (1986), The psychology of powerlessness. *Psychoanal. Inqu.*, 6:93–118.

Hamilton, J. W. (1978), Some remarks on certain vicissitudes of narcissism. *Internat. Rev. Psychoanal.* 5:275–284.

Hendrick, I. (1942), Instinct and the ego during infancy. *Psychoanal. Quart.*, 11:33–58.

Hobbes, T. (1651), *English Works*, Vol. 7. *Leviathan.* London: J. M. Dent, 1976.

Horner, A. J. (1996), *The Wish for Power and the Fear of Having It.* Northvale, NJ: Jason Aronson.

Howard, J. A., Blumstein, P., & Schwartz, P. (1986), Sex, power, and influence tactics in intimate relationships. *J. Person. & Soc. Psychol.*, 51:102–109.

Isay, R. A. (1980), Late adolescence: The second separation stage of adolescence. In: *The Course of Life: Psychoanalytic Contributions Toward Understanding Personality Development*, Vol. 11, ed. S. I. Greenspan & G. H. Pollock. Washington, DC: NIMH, pp. 511–522.

Kaplan, A. (1995), The power of culture. *Civilization*, September/October: 46–51. Washington, DC: The Library of Congress.

Kestenbaum. C. J. (1986), The professional woman's dilemma: Love and/or power. *Amer. J. Psychoanal.*, 46:15–21.

Klebanow, S. (1989), Power, gender and money. *J. Amer. Acad. Psychoanal.*, 17:321–328.

Kohut, H. (1966), Forms and transformations of narcissism. *J. Amer. Psychoanal. Assn.*, 14:243–272.

——— (1977), *The Restoration of the Self.* New York: International Universities Press.

——— (1985), On leadership. In: *Self Psychology and the Humanities: Reflections on a New Psychoanalytic Approach*, ed. C. B. Strozier. New York: W. W. Norton, pp. 51–72.

Lichtenberg, J. (1989), *Psychoanalysis and Motivation.* Hillsdale, NJ: Analytic Press.

Loewenberg, P. J. (1986), Nixon, Hitler, and power: An ego psychological study. *Psychoanal. Inqu.*, 6:27–48.

Mace, G. (1979), *Locke, Hobbes, and the Federalist Papers.* Carbondale: Southern Illinois University Press.

Machiavelli, N. (1513a), *The Prince*, tr. & ed. R. M. Adams. New York: W. W. Norton, 1992.

——— (1513b), *The Prince*, tr. & ed. Q. Skinner & R. Price. Cambridge, U.K.: Cambridge University Press, 1988.

McClelland, D. C. (1975), *Power—The Inner Experience.* New York: Irvington.

McNeill, W. H. (1984), *The Pursuit of Power.* Chicago: University of Chicago Press.

Mahler, M. (1965), On the significance of the normal separation–individuation phase. In: *Drives, Affects, Behavior*, Vol. 2, ed. M. Schur. New York: International Universities Press.

——— (1968), *On Human Symbiosis and the Vicissitudes of Individuation.* New York: International Universities Press.

———— Pine, F., & Bergman, A. (1975), *The Psychological Birth of the Human Infant.* New York: Basic Books.

Manchester, W. (1978), *American Caesar.* Boston: Little, Brown.

Nietzsche, F. (1886), *The Will to Power,* ed. W. Kaufmann, tr. W. Kaufmann & R. J. Hollingdale. New York: Random House, 1967.

Olsson, P. A. (1986), Complexities in the psychology and psychotherapy of the phenomenally wealthy. In: *The Last Taboo,* ed. D. W. Krueger. New York: Bruner/Mazel, pp. 53–69.

———— (1988), The terrorist and the terrorized, *J. Psychohist.,* 16:47–60.

Oremland, J. D. (1989), Michelangelo's Sistine Chapel Ceiling. *Applied Psychoanalysis Series,* Monogr. 2. Madison, CT: International Universities Press.

Parry, A. M. (1989), *The Language of Achilles and Other Papers.* Oxford: Clarendon Press.

Person, E. S. (1986), Male sexuality and power. *Psychoanal Inqu.,* 6:3–25.

Pine, F. (1985), *Developmental Theory and Clinical Process.* New Haven, CT: Yale University Press.

Plutarch (120–130 A.D.). Lives. *The Harvard Classics,* ed. C. W. Elliot. New York: P. F. Collier, 1909.

Raven, B. H. (1986), A taxonomy of power in human relations. *Psychiatric Ann.,* 16:633–636.

———— (1993), The bases of power: Origins and recent developments. *J. Soc. Iss.,* 49:227–251.

Rawlinson, M. C. (1987), Foucault's strategy. *J. Med. & Philosophy,* 12:371–395.

Robinson, C. E. (1916), *The Days of Alkibiades.* London: Edward Arnold.

Rousseau, J. J. (1762), *Social Contract.* Harmondsworth, U.K.: Penguin Books, 1968.

Russell, B. (1969), *Power, a New Social Analysis.* New York: W. W. Norton.

Shampo, M. A., & Kyle, R. A. (1982), Alexander the Great. *J. Amer. Psychoanal. Assn.,* 248:70.

Simon, B. (1986), The power of the wish and the wish for power: A discussion of power and psychoanalysis. *Psychoanal. Inqu.,* 6:119–131.

Smith, H. (1988), *The Power Game.* New York: Ballentine Books.

Springer, O., Ed. (1974), *Langenscheidt German-English Encyclopedia Dictionary.* Berlin: Langenscheidt Muret-Sanders.

Stern, D. N. (1977), *The First Relationship.* Cambridge, MA: Harvard University Press.

———— (1985), *The Interpersonal World of the Infant.* New York: Basic Books.

Strauss, L. (1984), *The Political Philosophy of Hobbes: Its Bases and Its Genesis.* Chicago: University of Chicago Press.

Syme, R. (1939), *The Roman Revolution.* Oxford: Oxford University Press, 1960.

———— (1963), *Tacitus.* 2 vols. Oxford: Clarendon Press.

Tacitus. Agricola and Germania. In: *Tacitus,* ed. T. A. Dorey. London: Routledge & Kegan Paul, 1969, pp. 1–18.

Tzu, Sun (c. 452–221 B.C.), *The Art of War,* ed. J. Clavell. New York: Dell/ Delta, 1983.

Waite, R. G. L. (1977), *The Psychopathic God: Adolph Hitler.* New York: Basic Books.

Winter, D. G. (1973), *The Power Motive.* New York: Free Press.

―――― (1987), Enhancement of an enemy's power motivation as a dynamic of conflict escalation. *J. Personal. & Soc. Psychol.,* 52:41–46.

Wrong, D. H. (1988), *Power, Its Forms, Bases and Uses.* Chicago: University of Chicago Press.

Young, D. (1960), *The Desert Fox.* New York: Berkley/Medalion.

Zimmermann, D. (1987), The institutional structures of psychoanalysis and their effects on the training of the analyst. *The Annual of Psychoanalysis,* 15:337–351. New York: International Universities Press.

Chapter 7

Narcissistic Rage in Young Adulthood: The Tragedy of Akhilleus

> Sing, Goddess, the anger of Peleus' Son Akhilleus
> and its devastation which put pains thousand fold
> upon the Achaians [Homer, *The Iliad,* I, 1–2].

In Richmond Lattimore's introduction to his translation of Homer's *Iliad* he states that this heroic poem is really "the story of Achilleus" (Lattimore, 1951, p. 17) and from his "anger of pride, the necessary accompaniment of the warrior's greatness, . . . springs the tragedy of the *Iliad*" (p. 47). It is my intention here to expand on this theme of anger; that is, traumatically overwhelming narcissistic rage. The Greek word is *menis* for vengeful *wrath* (Schein, 1984) felt by a god or a hero toward humans. In fact, Fagles (1990) translates it as *rage.*

Previous attempts at dealing with other literary figures who are depicted as afflicted with narcissistic rage are that of Melville's Captain Ahab in *Moby Dick* by Kligerman (1953), Kohut (1972), Hamilton (1978), and Gomez (1990); Heinrich von

Acknowledgment. When this paper was first conceived, I did not know of MacCary's (1982) book in which he posits a narcissistic theme in Akhilleus' behavior. I am indebted to Bennet Simon for directing my attention to this work.

I am choosing the classical spelling of Akhilleus rather than the Latinized version, Achilles.

181

Kleist's *Michael Kohlhaus* by Kohut (1972) and Dettmerling (1975); and George Eliot's Maggie in *The Mill on the Floss* by Johnstone (1990). I am indebted to all these authors for their groundbreaking work in this area of applied analysis concerning narcissistic rage since there is much to be learned from the novelist's attempts to depict the darker aspects of the human condition. Johnstone (1990), for example, described Maggie's low self-esteem that had resulted from her family's ongoing devaluation of her. She suicided when she realized there was no one who could possibly meet her needs for a mirroring selfobject. Gomez (1990) pointed out that Melville "used the magic of dreams, legends and myths to create a universally resonating great novel about one man's pride and obsession for revenge" (p. 64).

By pulling together the essential elements of the story that are pertinent to my thesis, I will show how Akhilleus's experiences from the present and the past in his life parallel the experiences of patients whose modern-day tragic lives required thoroughgoing psychoanalysis to gain control, resolution, and mastery over wounded pride, grandiose fantasies, and the traumatic experiences that led to their struggles with narcissistic rage. The mourning process (Freud, 1917) was especially crucial to progress in the analyses.

THE STORY OF AKHILLEUS

Akhilleus's ideals of justice, honor, and fair play led him to protest and insist that something had to be done to stop Apollo's retaliatory "silver arrows" (some sort of plague—*loinos*) that were devastating the Greek ranks. Apollo was upset with the Achaians for preventing his priest Chryses from rescuing his daughter Chryseis who had been taken by Agamemnon as a prize in an earlier raid. Akhilleus assembled the chieftains together to discuss what to do about this problem.

He implored:

> No, come, let us ask some holy man, some prophet,
> even an interpreter of dreams, since a dream also
> comes from Zeus, who can tell why Phoibos Apollo is so angry
> [1, 62–64].

Kalchas, the soothsayer, argued for giving the girl Chryseis back and Akhilleus supported him but this made Agamemnon furious—his

> heart within [is] filled black to the brim with anger from beneath, but his two eyes showed like fire in their blazing [1, 103–104].

Agamemnon yelled at Kalchas that if he had to give up his mistress, someone else had to give him their prize to replace her. Rebel that he was, Akhilleus called Agamemnon the "greediest for gain of all men" (1, 122) and that it was unfair and "unbecoming . . . for the people to call back things once given" (1, 126).

Agamemnon, stung by this contumacious impertinence from one of his soldiers, threatened to take Akhilleus's, Aias's or Odysseus's prize for himself. But Akhilleus was moved to retaliate with still another insult:

> O, wrapped in shamelessness, with your mind forever on profit how shall any one of the Achaians readily obey you either to go on a journey or to fight men strongly in battle? I for my part did not come here for the sake of the Trojan spearmen to fight against them, since to me they have done nothing
> [1, 149–153].

Akhilleus continued to attack Agamemnon by saying it wasn't his battle anyway, it was Agamemnon's and Menelaos's pride at stake. He was weary from having to bear the greater brunt of the battles, and besides, he always got the lesser portion of the war booty. So he thought he might just as well go home rather than remain to be dishonored, humiliated, and watch Agamemnon pile up his "wealth" and "luxury." Agamemnon didn't let Akhilleus get away with that. He retorted that Akhilleus was "the most hateful of all kings" and was "forever quarrelling" (1, 176–177).

Pulling rank, Agamemnon took Akhilleus's prize, a young woman called Briseis, for contending with him and to show him who was the greater man. Akhilleus was then terribly humiliated and publicly dishonored in front of his fellow Argives. In mounting rage, he escalated the argument as he called Agamemnon a greedy coward, a drunk, and he, Akhilleus, would be sorely missed in the coming battles. With that, he threw down the scepter. Suppressing his murderous rage, though, left him silently seething when he was stayed by Athene from running Agamemnon through with his sword. Nestor tried to mediate the quarrel, but the two adversaries merely hardened their positions following the same pattern as modern fathers' arguments with their sons when the fathers fail to understand the meaning of assertive adolescent behavior. Both parties often stubbornly refuse to listen to reason or each other.

Wise Odysseus pleaded with Akhilleus for the sake of friendship not to argue, and warned him of the anger of pride. Then Agamemnon got the last shot in by saying that Akhilleus was so grandiose as to wish for "power over all, and to be lord of all, and to give them their orders . . ." (1, 287–289).

The net result of this seemingly familiar generational controversy was that Akhilleus emerged the loser and was further embarrassed and humiliated. He felt helpless to do anything about the humiliation or the loss of his gift of honor (*geras*). He experienced *aidos*, translated as both shame and embarrassment by Cairns (1993). He withdrew to sulk in his tent like narcissistically traumatized patients and some adolescents characteristically do. He sought revenge by asking his goddess mother Thetis to intercede with Zeus to make it hard on the Greeks in the ensuing battles to make certain that his absence from the fray would be sorely missed. He wanted Agamemnon to suffer as much as he was suffering. He felt that he was being treated as a "dishonored vagabond" (1, 648). But, in my opinion, this dramatic situation was not just a generational or oedipal struggle. Rather, in this very competitive Greek society, the fight between the two men degenerated into more basic and profound narcissistic issues of shame, wounded pride, humiliation, helplessness, narcissistic injury, rage, and threatened loss of power and control on both sides (Kohut, 1985b). Cairns (1993) has suggested that Greek culture at the time emphasized the importance of shame (feeling abashed), because honor, glory, and reputation in battle were measured by the prizes or *geras* won in battle, although he believes guilt was also present in the warriors. Cairns believes, and I concur, that the difference between ancient Greece and modern Western society is "one of degree rather than of kind" (pp. 44–45). Even if the words were not there in the language, my reading of the culture is that they certainly felt both shame and guilt.

The young adult Akhilleus's personality as represented in the poem illustrates some of the issues common to late adolescents and young adults. These are phase specific tasks related to consolidation of the personality with an integration of a cohesive self or an intact identity; the development of a more benign superego and ego ideal; and reworking of the oedipal conflict as well as separation–individuation issues. However, as important as these issues are, not all of the conflict between Akhilleus and Agamemnon is understandable from that standpoint (Brockman, 1984).

The most telling issue in Akhilleus' struggle is a narcissistic rage that was mobilized by Agamemnon's insult in an already narcissistically injured self that seethed and simmered without respite. Furthermore, Akhilleus's withdrawal put him in a much more vulnerable situation while mourning (*akhos*) the loss of Briseis and his wounded pride and lowered self-esteem (Freud, 1917; Hägglund, 1975). Presumably, too, he had no other heterosexual outlet. But when his closest and only friend Patroklos was killed in battle while wearing Akhilleus's own armor (Shannon, 1975), he was even more devastated. He was then traumatically flooded by a new and more powerful process, that of mourning the loss of his best friend, a loss that he was totally unprepared for. He groaned like a lion (*achnutai*, King [1987]) "over his stolen cubs, [who] travels far in hopes of tracking down the hunter" (p. 20). Revenge would not let him rest until he had killed Hektor and brought his body and armor back to camp. Now he alone had to face his destiny on the wide plains of Troy. Neither did he have a family to console him, nor could he accept counsel from the wiser senior men in the expeditionary force. Additionally, with his own fate decided, his old father Peleus back at home would be left alone in his old age.

What was created was a more intense rage that was directed against himself, "against his own limited, finite, mortal human condition" (Sinaiko, 1981) and then redirected onto Hektor. I agree with Sinaiko's interpretation that Homer has thus breathed life into the greatest of all tragic figures in history in contrast to Redfield's (1975) contention that Hektor was the greater hero. Moreover, Sinaiko's claims that "Homer may be the only artist who measures up to Shakespeare" (1998, p. 39) is confirmed by the millions who have enjoyed this epic over the centuries and still do.

It appears that Akhilleus was possibly a young adolescent of about 14 when the Greek armada set sail for Troy (9, 458) but he must have been unusually large for his age. Puberty probably had already set in. Akhilleus was a boy king of the Myrmidons. He and all the other kings in the armada to Troy were former suitors of Helen who had sworn to defend her in case she was spirited away by someone. Since the poem begins nine years later, I am conjecturing that blond Akhilleus must have been in his late teens or early twenties, a young person whose entire adolescence had been spent away from home on the battlefields along the coasts of Asia Minor. Furthermore, he must have had a very imposing physique (18, 192–193). Aias, Patroklos, and Hecktor may have been of similar size, but the impression Homer gives is that Akhilleus was the largest of the warriors. Furthermore, just appearing on the barricades once without his armor, in addition to the fact that Athene "swept about his powerful shoulders the fluttering aegis" (18, 204) and crowned his head with a golden cloud of fire, was enough to frighten the Trojans into a "panicked disorder" so that twelve Trojans died. Thetis describes how fast he grew:

> . . . and he shot up like a young tree,
> and I nurtured him, like a tree grown
> in the pride of the orchard [18, 56–57].

His impressive size, his successes in battle, the help he repeatedly received from the gods, and the fame attributed to him and his Myrmidon troops contributed greatly to his arrogant illusion of grandiosity, not to speak of his disavowal of the knowledge of his foreshortened life. Also, he was deprived of the needed guidance and direction of caring, empathic parents during this critical adolescent rite of passage. Consolidation of his personality along adult lines was not yet completed. He pouted and sulked like a much younger person when he felt his prize Briseis was wrongfully taken away. But Agamemnon's behavior was no better, since he reacted to Akhilleus as a real rival, and failed to be the ideal mirroring parent surrogate and leader by lowering himself to Akhilleus's level. Moreover, Akhilleus was robbed of an idealized selfobject to merge with and to facilitate the second phase of separation-individuation as well as the more familiar adolescent working through of the oedipal conflict. Acting as though Akhilleus was a real rival parallels the common observation in modern-day patients whose fathers confirm the boy's worst fears of retaliatory castration when they regard their sons as real rivals. Humiliating shame (*aidos*) and threats of castration combined to produce a neurotic withdrawal in Akhilleus and in a similar way in Mr. R as described by Yorke (1990).

In addition, to complicate matters, Akhilleus threw away the respect of his peers. He withdrew to his tent. He played his lyre and sang of his past glories in a narcissistic withdrawal to comfort and soothe himself over the loss of Briseis and the public humiliation. How was he to regain honor, realize his ambitions, or live up to his own ideals of honor, fair play, and justice and regain self-respect by withdrawing and alienating himself from his peers? He was reduced to abject helplessness. The answer is, first, that it was through the natural growth-producing mourning and identification processes for his friend and alter ego Patroklos. Second, this was followed by the gradual rapprochement (Greenstadt, 1982) with his peers and later with Agamemnon, while renouncing bribes and greediness for material wealth.

Resolution of his rage, however, was not so easy to complete because Akhilleus's rage emanated from a deeper source that was easily transferred onto Hektor. When he returned to the battle, he killed with wild and ferocious abandon until he was covered with blood. He was virtually a killing machine. He truly was "beastly" (King, 1987). He had no mercy for young defenseless boys and Trojan warriors alike. In a fit of grandiosity, he even defied the river Skamandros's torrents and was almost drowned except for Hephaistos's intervention of a wall of fire to tame the river. He was really transformed into something demonic, and was compared to a ferocious lion.

This overpowering rage is not to be confused with the so-called adaptive aggression of modern soldiers who are motivated by the realistic dangers of battle (Fox, 1974). On the other hand, homicidal adolescents today, according to McCarthy (1978), are "characterized by a vengeful narcissistic rage expressed through violent acts as attacks on a poorly integrated part-self-object" (p. 21). Furthermore, he indicated that "deprivation and rejection by early objects provide the framework for narcissistic disturbances in homicidal adolescents" (p. 21). Akhilleus was clearly in a rage that appeared to have no end. Some measure of his rage against Agamemnon was taken when Akhilleus said: "no, not if his gifts outnumbered all the grains of sand and dust in the earth" (Fagles, 9, 470–471). All the opulent gifts promised by Agamemnon were he to return to battle were refused outright. He said he couldn't fight for such a self-serving leader as Agamemnon. He realized, though, his fate was sealed. If he returned home, he would live but the glory and honor of victory in battle would be denied him. If he stayed, he knew he had to die. He was caught in a monumental dilemma that heightened the drama. A solution was presented to him when Patroklos begged to enter the fight. He gave Patroklos his inherited, special armor that had been given to Peleus by the Uranian gods and sent him into battle as an alter ego.

MYTHOLOGICAL CONSIDERATIONS

What is it then in Akhilleus's mythological background (Graves, 1955, pp.305–334) that would give rise to such an extraordinary response to what started out as a common soldiers' quarrel and ended up as a major event? First of all, Larousse's *Mythology* (1959) states that Akhilleus's mother, the Nereid goddess Thetis herself, was humiliated by being betrothed to a mortal man, Peleus, even though he was a great warrior who had traveled with the Argonauts. Also, Peleus's father was Aiakos, the son of Zeus. Thetis and Peleus had seven sons, the first six of whom she threw into the fire, while Thetis is said to have been very tender to her seventh son, Akhilleus. However, one source (Appollonios) described Peleus's horror when he saw Thetis also putting Akhilleus in the fire, ostensibly to make him immortal. Peleus grabbed the screaming baby from her as she ran out, abandoning the baby. Peleus turned the care of the child over to Cheiron. In the more familiar version, she immersed him in the river Styx. His body then was supposed to be protected from harm save for the heel with which she held him in the water. In the *Iliad*, however, there is no mention of the vulnerable heel, except for the fact that everyone knows about it. Cheiron added to the myth of Akhilleus's invincibility by feeding him the marrowbones of bears and the entrails of lions as well as teaching him Aesculapian skills. In the *Iliad* he is said to have been nurtured mainly by Phoinix who raised him from infancy to be a "speaker of words and a doer of deeds" (A. M. Parry, 1989, p. 4). Phoinix held him on his lap while feeding him pieces of meat and wine, and we are told Akhilleus spat up on Phoinix's shirt (9, 486–491). His mother Thetis was not the attentive nurturing mother (and here I differ with MacCary, 1982) since she had abandoned him as a child and left to associate with the gods on Olympos and most of the time resided in her cave under the sea.

When he was 9 Kalchas predicted that Akhilleus alone would conquer Troy, but Thetis foresaw that her son would prematurely meet death on the wide plains of Troy, and tried to save him by hiding him in Lycomedes' castle dressed as a girl, a humiliation in itself. But when Odysseus planned a mock raid, Akhilleus was tricked and unmasked and was thus conscripted into the expeditionary force. Later on, when his armor (all except the Pelean ash spear that Akhilleus alone could wield) was taken by Hektor from Patroklos's corpse, Athene arranged for the god Hephaistos to forge him another impressive set. He was mortal but also a demigod, being the son of a goddess, the son of a hero who had brought back the Golden Fleece, and the grandson of Zeus. His horses were the fastest of all, having been given to his father Peleus by Poseidon. All these divine interventions, I think, served to give the mythic character of Akhilleus the grandiose illusion of immortality and invincibility (Burkert, 1979). But abandonment in infancy left a massive narcissistic scar that was reactivated by the public humiliation of the loss of Briseis and the recognition of his less than godlike human condition.

As the tragedy unfolded, however, Akhilleus entered into a process of resolution and reparation. The first indication of this was when he heard that Agamemnon, Diomedes, and Odysseus had been wounded. This was truly divine justice and a soothing satisfaction to his vengeful heart. Furthermore, he was forced to accept the inevitability that all humans suffer and die when his dearest and closest friend (alter ego or self-selfobject) Patroklos was killed while wearing Akhilleus's special armor (Shannon, 1975). Identification with Patroklos, who was the gentlest and kindest of all the heroes, began to take place. Momentarily, he toyed with the idea of reconciling with Agamemnon. Van Brock (1959) suggested that Patroklos was an alterego ("un autre soi-meme") in her linguistic studies of ritual substitutes in ancient Greek and Hittite poetry.

But his rage was not so easily set aside, and it was readily displaced onto Hektor. He showed no mercy in pursuing the enemy and finally running Hektor through with his spear. The "mutilation of the corpse theme" (Segal, 1971), by dragging Hektor's body behind his chariot about the battlefield, and three more times around Patroklos's bier, was the ultimate horrifying revenge, but at the same time it was unquenching compensation for his continuing savage rage. He even threatened to cut up and eat Hektor's raw flesh.

While at first resisting his grief, he slowly began to mourn the loss of Patroklos. After receiving Thetis's promise that Patroklos's body wouldn't deteriorate and the visitation of Patroklos's shade (*eidolon*) in a dream pleading for burial, Akhilleus experienced a growing release from his wrath and called for a major celebration of athletic games to honor his dead friend. The funeral rites also initiated a release for the processes of grief and mourning. "Achilleus has broken out of the self-imposed prison of godlike unrelenting fury, reintegrated himself in society, returned to something like human feeling; he is part of the community again" (Fagles, 1990, p. 58).

He now acknowledged the fact he couldn't control the gods or the conditions of war. Slowly but surely, he came to recognize his need for other people. Aphrodite's and Apollo's protection of Hektor's body from deterioration paralleled the protection of Patroklos's body. As he acquiesced to the gods' criticism and their injunction to release the corpse, his wrath was spent. Akhilleus, then, reversed his alienation from his comrades-in-arms. Most importantly, he was deeply touched by the profound and eloquently spoken grief of Priam when Priam grasped his knees and begged for the return of his son Hektor's body. The courage, too, that Priam showed in coming alone to the Greek camp was impressive to our hero. Akhilleus was then faced with the task of working through the helplessness and humiliation that precipitated his narcissistic rage. First, he felt pity and then love for his own father, his own son Neoptolemos back in Skyros (19, 325–327), and finally for Priam who had lost many more sons in addition to Hektor. In effect, he resonated and empathized with Priam's grief. The two men even admired each other. Akhilleus fed Priam a feast and put him up for the night, confirming a profound rapprochement. Affirming his commitment to higher ideals and values and the conversion of pathological arrogance and infantile grandiosity into empathy for the grieving father, helped him to forge a more adult ego ideal structure. A stronger sense of reality and self-esteem returned. Furthermore, as Lattimore has described Akhilleus as an intelligent gentleman of nobility and culture, we observe that those characteristics were restored when he presided over the athletic games and entertained friends. Thus, pathological narcissistic strivings (Kohut, 1966) were partially transformed through the mourning of Patroklos and the emergence of empathy for Priam's loss of his son Hektor. It must be remembered that Akhilleus was also a healer, having learned the art of healing from Aesculapius and Patroklos.

There is some merit to MacCary's (1982) thesis here that Akhilleus's self is actualized after both selfobjects—Patroklos and Hektor—are dead. But my contribution here is that the mourning process was what facilitated the transformation of narcissistic rage and the reinstatement of an arrested developmental process of acquiring an adult form of ego ideal and a healthy management of grandiose fantasy. Snell (1905) suggests internal dialogue is absent in Homeric mental life, but the thesis here is the contrasting view that a developmental process is partially actualized by interventions of the gods, but more so by the healing of an internal narcissistic injury. In literary terms, the ritualistic substitution of a formerly savage sacrificial object so that an important object can live is "poetized" in the *Iliad* (Van Brock, 1959).

Homer has depicted both the horrors and the glory of war in an unsentimental manner devoid of moralizing in his effort to present the "beauty, the rewards, and the price of human heroism" (Schein, 1984, p. 84). However, Simone Weil, motivated by the horrors of the Holocaust in World War II, emphasized in her magnificent essay that might is not the answer and "the understanding of human suffering is dependent on justice, and love is its condition" (1977, p. 181). Moreover, one could say that in the *Iliad* ideals, after all, can contribute to a kind of virtuous triumph in the end!

The story of Akhilleus is a model for us clinically as well as from the literary point of view. Knox says in his notes to Fagles (1990), "Homer's Achilles is clearly the model for the tragic hero of the Sophoclean stage; his stubborn, passionate devotion to an ideal image of the self is the same force that drives Antigone, Oedipus, Ajax and Philoctetes to the fulfillment of their destinies" (Fagles, 1990, p. 63). He is indeed the "best of the Achaians" (1,244,412;16,274). He is "preeminent in beauty, swiftness, strength, and all-around fighting ability as well as in his horses and armor" (Schein, 1984, p. 91). He was the most complex of heroes. Even his shield depicted contrasting scenes of war and peace, blood price and wedding dances, the grape harvest and lions attacking herds of sheep in a pastoral meadow.

THEORETICAL CONSIDERATIONS

Kohut (1972) has indicated that narcissistic rage occurs when a narcissistically vulnerable person responds to an actual or expected narcissistic injury. This rage is precipitated by experiences of being the object of "ridicule, contempt, or conspicuous defeat." It takes the form of "the need for revenge, for righting a wrong, for undoing a hurt by whatever means, and a deeply anchored unrelenting compulsion in pursuit of all these aims which gives no rest to those who have suffered a narcissistic injury—these are features which are characteristic for the phenomena of narcissistic rage in all its forms and which set it apart from all other kinds of aggression" (p. 380). The intellect is sharpened and is turned to the task of seeking sweet revenge and retribution. It is rooted in the "uncompromising insistence in the perfection of the idealized selfobject and on the limitlessness of the power and knowledge of a grandiose self" (p. 385). In contrast, realistic mature aggressions are limited. Kohut indicated that narcissistic rage:

> [A]rises when self or object fail to live up to the absolutarian expectations which are directed at their function—whether by a child who more or less phase-appropriately, insists on the grandiosity and omnipotence of the self and the selfobject or by the narcissistically fixated adult whose archaic narcissistic structures have remained unmodified because they became isolated from the growing psyche after the phase appropriate narcissistic demands of childhood had been traumatically frustrated [p. 386].

He goes on to say that narcissistic rage occurs when there is a failure of the "unconditional availability of the approving mirroring functions of an admiring selfobject or on the ever-present opportunity for a merger with an idealized one" (p. 386). What is also posited here is that a fragmentation of the self occurs as a result of the narcissistic injury. Galatzer-Levy (1993) pointed out that violence in the adolescent is due to a desperate effort to maintain or restore an endangered or fragmenting self. Robertiello (1976) emphasized what Freud had pointed out earlier in "Mourning and Melancholia" (1917) regarding the narcissistic loss of self-esteem from object loss. Hägglund (1975) reiterated Freud's point that the loss of an object is a narcissistic one, and the mourning is made all the more difficult for the more narcissistic person. One is reminded here also of Bibring's contribution (1953) about the mechanism of depression when he described the ego's response of helplessness to a real or imaginary loss by diminished self-esteem and a flooding of the ego with unmanageable affect.

Terman (1975) amplified Kohut's thesis with a clinical example of a woman whose core trauma was her father's frustrating failure to respond appropriately to her needs for merger with the omnipotent selfobject and with appropriate affect to her as an oedipal girl. There was exposure to family nudity and the father was unduly harsh with inferiors and was quite bigoted. Transmuting internalizations led to her enhanced capacity to internalize the good analyst that served to heal the injured self.

Wolf (1988) devoted an entire chapter in his book to narcissistic rage. He emphasized unendurable helplessness vis-à-vis the humiliating selfobject parent. "Such experiences are so traumatic because they threaten the very continuity and existence of the self and they therefore evoke the strongest emergency defense of the self . . ." (p. 80). In Wolf's experience, narcissistic rage is manifest as homicidal or suicidal fantasies and is associated with intolerable helplessness. Rage smolders inside and reemerges from its position lurking beneath the surface when the integrity of the self is threatened by some real or perceived, destructive, destabilizing insult. Dodes (1990) also emphasized the sense of helplessness and focused on what he called an "addictive vulnerability" of persons with self-deficits. Many Vietnam veterans were addicted to various drugs and alcohol that they used to medicate their impending fragmentation and narcissistic rage. McCarthy (1978) described homicide in adolescents as a defense against further disintegration of the personality already beset with severe fragmentation. Marohn (1991) described narcissistic rage as occurring in certain personalities along a continuum from a very primitive pole to a more structured pole. He presented a group of observations from his work with adolescents who experienced severe trauma in childhood.

Fox (1974) described the differences between narcissistic rage and adaptive combat aggression in Vietnam veterans, and Parson (1984) discussed the repair processes of the self in therapeutic work with Vietnam veterans who had suffered severe posttraumatic stress disorder.

Arlow (1961, 1991) used ego psychological concepts while Greenstadt (1982) used Mahler's theory of separation-individuation to amplify and explain the clinical phenomena of personal and ancient myths as well as the uses of myths in cultures and societies. Schore (1991, 1992) traced the onset of humiliating shame to overstimulation during the practicing subphase of development when the child who excitedly is expecting to share some charged affective state with the mother but who experiences instead a massive "misattunement, thereby triggering a sudden shock-induced deflation of affect" (1991, pp. 187–188). An entire issue of the *Bulletin of the Menninger Clinic* (1994) was devoted to the clinical study of the effects of traumatic humiliation in childhood.

MacCary posited an "Achilles Complex" created by an all-loving and all-giving mother who is always present. However, in my reading of the poem, Thetis wasn't so available. He borrows heavily from the philosophy of Hegel and Lacan's psychoanalytic approach to support his views of the narcissistic problem in Akhilleus. Though his arguments are very scholarly and intellectually persuasive, they are seriously lacking in clinical relevance or authenticity. Narcissistic rage, then, arises in a narcissistically vulnerable person when his self-esteem is so injured by maternal deprivation as to induce an overwhelming sense of helplessness and anger. Such persons enjoy no relief from the suffering they experience even when revenge is realized. Further personality growth is not possible. The traumatically injured and fragmented self has to be healed through transmuting experiences in the transference with an empathically understanding selfobject. A more classical theoretical approach suggests that a regressive process ensues resulting in a negative oedipal transference conflict combined with issues of separation-individuation. Reversal of the regression and resolution of the conflicts can emerge, however, when certain real-life events such as the mourning process provide the opportunity for change. But it goes without saying that the possibilities for change are most favorable in a psychoanalytic setting.

The oedipal conflict in Akhilleus, and in some patients, deserves appropriate attention because the triangular nature of the conflict is patently obvious. Competition for the prize Briseis and losing that battle certainly conforms to a classical triangular conflict, and Akhilleus experienced defeat at the hands of a perceived superior adversary who was the leader of the armada. But it is the very nature of Akhilleus's response of unrelenting anger and revenge from overwhelming shaming humiliation that leads me to say that Akhilleus's rage (and in my patient) was primarily narcissistic. It is true, as I have pointed out (1984), that oedipal conflicts as well as separation–individuation issues are being reworked in the late adolescent phase and continue on into young adulthood. But it is the uncompromising, paralyzing qualities of narcissistic rage, its origins and consequences, that deserve to be elaborated. Shame is phenomenonologically and theoretically different from guilt (Schore, 1992). Shame is related more to humiliation, mortification, remorse, apathy, embarrassment, and lowered self-esteem (Morrison, 1983). Piers and Singer (1971) make similar distinctions. Rudolph (1981) reported the case of a 10-year-old boy who had been put in a body cast from age 3 to 18 months. A five-year analysis resulted in the transformation of narcissistic rages into normal aggression, humor, and caring for others.

THE CASE OF MR. R

The analytic termination phase in a patient had been immediately preceded by a set of issues that dealt with a deep-seated sense of shame and humiliation that we traced to the overstimulating, rejecting parents who had repeatedly pointed out his failures to measure up to their expectations. He felt helpless to restore his sense of self-esteem, while the only bright spot in his past was a loving grandparent who served as an important transference source in the analysis. As these early conflictual issues with his parents, along with the later oedipal issues, were repeatedly interpreted and worked through, he felt freer and stronger to make friends with and associate with both men and women with different educational backgrounds without feeling inferior and ashamed. He developed a more adult ego ideal and a more benign superego. He learned to cope with and modulate his primitive, passionate nature and enjoyed a strengthening of a modulating and flexible ego that was relatively resistant to regression and the previously stereotypical drivenness of an imperious rage. Acceptance of the transience of life, an increasing wisdom about what life brings, and relations between people were matched by caring for others and a delightful sense of humor. He gained control of his emotions and especially his rage. He became a loving adult husband to his wife, a very attentive father to his children, and sensitive to their individual needs and feelings. He no longer engaged in the provocative adolescent transference behavior that was characteristic of the early part of the analysis. He was quietly grateful for the benefits of the analysis and confident the future would be bright. In a word, he transformed his rage into useful energies to conduct his work that had been such a struggle for him before. A sturdy superego was fashioned that was much more benign, gentle, and kind. The ego ideal turned into a functionally intact complementary structure that served him well at work, at home, and at play. Involvement with his religious faith was integrated with the results of our analytic work. He was grateful for the result that he had longed for over so many years of his life.

Another clinical instance of narcissistic rage proved to be amenable to psychoanalytic treatment. Mr. T came to treatment when the breakup of his marriage was imminent. He was very anxious and had been a heavy drinker until shortly before entering analysis. The drinking had stopped but at the expense of a severely constricted personality. He was remote and totally absorbed with his inner life that was in turmoil.

What emerged from our genetic constructions of Mr. T's early childhood was that his father was unmercifully humiliating to him on every occasion when he attempted to assert himself. The only comfort he encountered was clinging to his depressed mother and watching her nude body as she moved from the bath to the bedroom to get dressed. He remained in a very low-level position in his occupational field avoiding the expected humiliating criticism that he had been subjected to in childhood and adolescence. Even though he had completed a master's degree with high marks from a prestigious Midwestern university, he was unable to make use of his superior intellect until he had repeated and worked through in the transference much of the humilating circumstances that had given rise to narcissistic rage and intense fantasies of sadistic violent revenge. The Oedipus complex was complicated by the fact that his father had perceived and interacted with him as a real rival. A sensitively positive empathic therapeutic alliance relationship allowed him to reveal his pain and rage and reenact it in the transference. He developed a stronger sense of self-esteem and is now able to use his many intellectual gifts in mathematical as well as literary areas. For example, he enjoyed solving complicated calculus and physics problems while deriving the formulae in his solutions. His intellectual interests are protean including anthropology and astronomy and he loves to entertain his friends by reciting emotionally moving, lengthy passages from the great poets in English literature. He has developed a warm and charming sociable persona that endears him to men and women alike.

In another clinical example of narcissistic rage, a father became enraged when his son had the temerity to question him about a domestic dispute. Prior to this event, they had enjoyed the closest of relationships, including hiking and camping trips to exotic places in the world. To raise doubts about the father's motives and behavior in the dispute was so intolerable that he did not speak to the son for a year. But the pain of the alienation and loss of what had been such a close relationship led the father to seek psychotherapy.

SUMMARY

The onset of a narcissistic rage is related to the experience of traumatic humiliating shame in early childhood and adolescence (Greenacre, 1952). Clinical experience with this problem is amenable to psychoanalysis when the deeply repressed and affect laden memories of repeated humiliations are uncovered and worked through in the transference. Both Mr. R and Mr. T were highly motivated to root out the traumatic experiences of childhood that had laid down a wellspring of combative rage. The added factor of both fathers reacting and relating to their sons as though they were real rivals complicated the transference. Furthermore, in both clinical instances cited, there was overstimulation from exposure to family nudity in early childhood. The in-depth study of Homer's characterization of Akhilleus paralleled and resembled what is described in the clinical cases cited.*

APPENDIX

*Several questions arise about Homer's poem: What is so unique about this story? Why has this legend been so attractive, so endearing, and so fascinating to scores of readers over the ages? Is it meeting Matthew Arnold's criteria (as cited in Lattimore's Introduction, 1951, p. 55) for the perfect translation that must be faithful to Homer's plainness in diction, style and thought; simple in ideas; flowingly rapid in movement; noble in manner; and possessing a smoothness of the hexameter that is free of "fancifulness" (Arnold, 1905)? Is it the discovery of the most essential elements of the human mind (Snell, 1905)? Or is it, as Simon (1978) suggests, that this kind of heroic poetry appeared at a time when heroes were "gone and their absence is mourned" (p. 53)? I think yes to both Arnold and Simon. In this same connection, Rohde's thesis (1898) is that the "cult of heroes was a highly evolved transformation of the worship of ancestors" (Nagy, 1990, p. 11). Another answer would be the creative and poetic use of such linguistic structures as symmetry (Schein, 1984) and imagery; the linguistic use of the noun-epithet and conjunction–verb formulae and the process of enjambment (M. Parry, 1971); and metaphor (Blackwell, 1735) as well as simile (Sinaiko, 1981, 1998) that add literary color and charm to the story. Second, the brutal, cruel, and horrible aspects of an action-filled war are made more tolerable to the reader by the dramatic device of juxtapositioning the human, peacetime scenes alongside that of the gory battlefield (Lattimore, Introduction, 1951; Sinaiko, 1981). Third, it is the history of a whole culture (Bury, 1913; Kraft, Kayan, and Erol, 1980; M. Wood, 1985) being recalled in terms of a romantic epic (M. Parry, 1971) and the earliest known written Western literature of mankind (Sinaiko, 1998). Fourth, it is a creative opportunity to project one's own issues (Arlow, 1961, 1991) onto the noble but human, fallible, and tragically alienated character (Kohut, 1977), personal fate or destiny (*Moira*) (Greenstadt, 1982) of Akhilleus who succumbed to a narcissistic rage. Fifth, and in a related sense, Homer's tragic poetry was and still is a kind of catharsis therapy, originally stated by Aristotle (Simon, 1978, p. 47). The result is a relieving affective discharge of the tensions generated by the poem (J. Bernays, 1857, as cited in *Freud's Women*, L. Appignanesi and J. Forrester, 1992, p. 28). Finally, Homer has combined in Akhilleus's character a "critique of heroic society [with] his exploration of what it means to be human, mortal" (King, 1987, p.

1). Cool reason and "starts of passion" (Blackwell, 1735) are combined in Homer's mythical poetry. Burkert (1979, p. 1) asserts in his Sather Lectures that myths are a traditional narrative that are used as a designation for some part of reality. A myth is an applied narrative describing a meaningful and important reality that refers to the aggregate and going beyond the individual. Tragedies are very attractive and appealing to audiences, and, according to Aristotle, the essential element of tragedy is an imitation not so much of persons but of their actions and their lives in the form of misery or happiness (*Poetics*, 6:16–17). The *Iliad* is indeed a classical tragedy full of action and is accompanied by much misery as well as happiness! Aristotle also declared that tragedy is composed of six parts: namely "Spectacle, Character, Fable (or Plot), Diction, Melody and Thought." The plot comes first and the characters are second like the colors on a painting, and they give a moral sense (*Poetics*, 6:39–41). Kohut's (1985a) view is that tragedy is "a repeatable, and thus dosed, experience. It allows us, therefore, to participate in the emotional development of the tragic hero from doubt to decision and from dejection to triumph as his nuclear self attains realization and is made permanent through death. Paradoxically, the spectator, participating in the ultimate self-realization of the tragic hero, experiences his own self as more vigorous and cohesive than he ever can in his real life" (p. 39).

Finally, the poem's appeal resides in the special admixture of Akhilleus's extraordinary, heroic (*aristeia*) physical prowess, his aristocratic superior qualities of personal greatness and before it was too late, the near complete resolution of his pathological rage by the mourning process of reparation (Klein, 1948). Akhilleus was truly the "best of the Achaians" (Nagy, 1979) in that he was the swiftest, most beautiful, youngest, and most complex (King, 1987). He was a fierce killer-warrior, but he alone played the lyre and sang of his past deeds. However artful, this was part of his narcissistic withdrawal to soothe and comfort himself for the blows to his self-esteem. In him are united "the extreme polarities of Homer's heroic world, which are also in part the polarities of all Greek culture: immense capacities for love and for hatred, social responsibility and self centered recklessness, devotion to personal ties and tragic isolation" (Segal, 1971, p. ix). *Arete* is merit or ability and achievement and is not a moral property but consists of nobility, achievement, success and reputation (Snell, 1905, p. 158). Moreover, the *Iliad* is replete with multiple opposites such as praise and blame (Nagy, 1990), shame and guilt versus honor and glory and high ideals versus brutal warfare.

Psychoanalytically speaking, the poem is about the psychological development of an idealized heroic self from a barbaric overgrown adolescent marauder to a godlike young adult proponent of the highest ideals. What [M. Parry] "found in Homer was not only the romantic possibility of a poetry expressive of a whole people, but also a quality of purposive directness which spoke strongly to the artistic sense of his own time" (A. Parry, 1989, p. 218). Akhilleus was assisted from time to time by the gods and in fact, the actions of all men were ultimately determined by the gods, how the battles were won or lost, and yet the gods were conceived to be subject to the same laws of the cosmos as humans are, besides being petty, quarreling and duplicitous.

Similarly, one patient was exquisitely inspired by the Christian Trinity and strove to follow the guidance of God the Father, God the Son, and the Holy Spirit. He prayed for divine assistance in following God's will. He firmly believed that he had been "led" to contact me as his therapist because as it turned out the analytic relationship was an especially good fit that he characterized as the most perfect one possible. In every aspect of his life, he strove to achieve perfection, similar to Akhilleus, and he held very strong views about justice, honor, and the right way to do things. His self-esteem had suffered from many severe woundings of his pride in the past that he was unable to heal by himself. Intense shame was the result (Lynd, 1958). He was militantly competitive and when his brother died at an early age like his father, he was faced with his own mortality, just as Akhilleus was when his best friend Patroklos was killed. Also, another parallel with Akhilleus was that several patients were severely narcissistically wounded as children that made them vulnerable to later real or imagined insults and humiliations.

In Homer, "virtue" and "good" mean to realize one's nature and one's wishes for perfection. In fact, Snell (1905) thinks there are three motivations for virtue in Homer: profit, search for happiness, and a drive for achievement, glory, and immortality that surpasses other nobles (Achaians). Certain positive aspects of Akhilleus's literary personality were so tragically marred by the distortion and miscarriage of his ideals, of compassion (*philotes*), humaneness, honor (*time*), loyalty, fairplay, and justice that deteriorated into unrelenting, unforgiving, irrational strivings for wrathful (*menis*) revenge even if it meant death to his comrades-in-arms. We can identify, resonate, and in a word empathize with the tragedy of Akhilleus. He is a hero because we can feel for him and his wounded pride and shame have meaning for us today. We would like to be like him when he is glorious and we can suffer with him because his human vulnerability—his narcissistic rage—is familiar to us as clinicians and as humans. Getting in touch with patients' narcissistic rage can be very trying and difficult clinically but when the right fit can occur much progress can be made. One particular patient was just as likeable and evocative of empathy as is Akhilleus to the modern reader.

The achievement of control and curbing of the passions was what Socrates called *sophrosyne*. Snell (1905) calls this factor of moderation "a moral measure, designed to stabilize the harmony of a healthy life" (p. 184). North (1966), however, declares that in the heroic age of the *Iliad* and the *Odyssey*, *sophrosyne* "is devoid of moral and religious implications; in three of the four passages it clearly denotes 'prudence or shrewdness' in one's own interest . . ." (p. 3). For my patients, however, it was both a moral and psychoanalytic victory to moderate and master their rage. They developed a more loving, kinder, and wiser disposition toward others.

In a general way, the processes some patients traversed to gain control, moderate, and overcome, or in more accurate psychoanalytic language transcend, transmute, and transform significant aspects of their narcissistic rage, follow a mourning process that was stimulated by the loss of an unfulfilled relationship with a parent and in the termination phase mourning the analytic relationship (Klein, 1948).

Finally, from the literary standpoint, I am following Norman Holland's (1968, 1975) thesis of responding to the affective contents of Homer's epic poem in a way similar to what a clinician does with clinical data. Holland's thesis essentially is locating a "central theme . . . that unifies an entire human personality" (p. 258).

Whitman (1958), Gouldner (1965), Slater (1968), Segal (1971), MacCary (1982), Snell (1905), and King (1987) have attempted to bring psychological meaning to Akhilleus's wrath, all of whom deserve to be studied with care. Slater (1968) and Gouldner (1965), for example, contended the Greeks in the *Iliad* were a quarrelsome lot and were unusually preoccupied with issues of fame, pride, and grandiosity (p. 4). There was much physical vanity and they were preoccupied "with honor, and glory"—*kleos*—(p. 35). In fact, Akhilleus was willing "to trade a long uneventful life for a brief one filled with honor and glory" (p. 35). Slater (1968) traces this narcissistic psychopathology to the ambivalent mother—son relationship where the "most grandiose self-definitions are at once fomented and punctured" (p. 44). Gouldner emphasizes the sociocultural aspects of Akhilleus's quarrel, *neikos*, with Agamemnon. He constructs the Homeric epic as a picture of that violent competitive society, the aim of which was to put another man down and to be autonomous. This was the tension between Akhilleus and Agamemnon. Agamemnon's power rested in the fact of his higher social rank and that he provided the most men and ships while Akhilleus's existed in his prowess in battle (Gouldner, 1965, pp. 13–14). There is a parallel quarrel between Akhilleus and Odysseus. My patient resembled those heroic Greeks in that he had to be the best in everything and he was as quarrelsome with just about everyone including me in the transference.

The archaeological findings of Kraft, Kayan, and Erol (1980) substantiate some of the descriptions of the terrain in the poem.

REFERENCES

Appignanesi, L., & Forrester, J. (1992), *Freud's Women.* New York: Basic Books.

Appollonios of Rhodes (1929), *Argonautica,* ed. R. C. Seaton. Oxford: Oxford University Press.

Aristotle, Poetics. In: *The Basic Works of Aristotle.* New York: Random House, 1946.

Arlow, J. A. (1961), Ego psychology and the study of mythology. *J. Amer. Psychoanal. Assn.,* 9:371–393.

———— (1991), The personal myth. In: *The Personal Myth in Psychoanalytic Theory,* ed. P. Hartocollis & I. D. Graham. Madison, CT: International Universities Press, pp. 21–35.

Arnold, M. (1905), *On Translating Homer.* New York: Ams Press.

Bibring. E. (1953), The mechanism of depression. In: *Affective Disorders,* ed. P. Greenacre. New York: International Universities Press, pp. 15–48.

Blackwell, T. (1735), *An Enquiry into the Life and Writings of Homer.* London.

Brockman, D. D., Ed. (1984), *Late Adolescence: Psychoanalytic Studies.* New York: International Universities Press.

Bulletin of the Menninger Clinic (1994), Fear of humiliation: Integrated treatment of social phobia and comorbid conditions. Vol. 58, Suppl. A.

Burkert, W. (1979), *Structure and History: Greek Mythology and Ritual.* Berkeley: University of California Press.

Bury, J. B. (1913), *A History of Greece.* New York: Random House/Modern Library.

Cairns, D. L. (1993), *Adios, The Psychology and Ethics of Honor and Shame in Ancient Greek Literature.* Oxford: Clarendon Press.

Dettmerling, P. (1975), The psychodynamics of Kleist's Michael Kohlhaus. *Psyche,* 29:154–170.

Dodes, L. M. (1990), Addiction, helplessness, and narcissistic rage. *Psychoanal. Quart.,* 59:398–419.

Fagles, R. (1990), *Homer: The Iliad,* ed. B. Knox. New York: Viking Press.

Fox, R. P. (1974), Narcissistic rage and the problem of combat aggression. *Arch. Gen. Psychiatry,* 31:807–811.

Freud, S. (1917), Mourning and melancholia. *Standard Edition,* 14:237–258. London: Hogarth Press, 1957.

Galatzer-Levy, R. M. (1993), Adolescent violence and the adolescent self. *Adol. Psychiatry,* 19:418–441. Chicago: University of Chicago Press.

Gomez, E. A. (1990), The Narcissus legend, the white whale, and Ahab's narcissistic rage: A self-psychological perspective. *J. Amer. Acad. Psychoanal.,* 18:644–653.

Gouldner, A. W. (1965), *Enter Plato.* New York: Basic Books.

Graves, R. (1955), *The Greek Myths.* Mt. Kisco, NY: Moyer Bell.

Greenacre, P. (1952), *Trauma, Growth and Personality.* New York: W. W. Norton.

Greenstadt, W. M. (1982), Heracles: A heroic figure of the rapprochement crisis. *Internat. Rev. Psychoanal.,* 9:1–23.

Hägglund, T-B. (1975), Mourning and narcissism. *Psychiatria Fennica.* pp. 151–156.

Hamilton, J. W. (1978), Some remarks on certain vicissitudes of narcissism. *Internat. Rev. Psychoanal.,* 5:275–284.

Holland, N. N. (1968), *The Dynamics of Literary Response.* New York: Oxford University Press.

——— (1975), *Readers Reading.* New Haven, CT: Yale University Press.

Homer (1920), *Homeri Opera,* ed. D. B. Munro & T. W. Allen, 5 vols. London: Oxford Classical Texts.

——— *The Iliad of Homer,* ed. & tr. R. Lattimore. Chicago: University of Chicago Press, 1951.

Johnstone, P. R. F. (1990), Narcissistic rage in the *Mill on the Floss. Lit. & Psychol.,* 26:90–109.

King, K. C. (1987), *Achilles: Paradigms of the War Hero from Homer to the Middle Ages.* Berkeley: University of California Press.

Klein, M. (1948), *Contributions to Psychoanalysis.* London: Hogarth Press.

Kligerman, C. (1953), The psychology of Herman Melville. *Internat. Psychoanal.,* 40:125–143.

Kohut, H, (1966),Forms and transformations of narcissism. *J. Amer. Psychoanal. Assn.*, 14:243–272.

—————— (1972), Narcissism and narcissistic rage. In: *The Psychoanalytic Study of the Child*, 27:360–400. Chicago: Quadrangle.

—————— (1977), *The Restoration of the Self.* New York: International Universities Press.

—————— (1985a), On courage. In: *Self Psychology and the Humanities: Reflections on a New Psychoanalytic Approach*, ed. R. Strozier. New York: W. W. Norton, pp. 5–50.

—————— (1985b), On leadership. In: *Self Psychology and the Humanities: Reflections on a New Psychoanalytic Approach*, ed. R. Strozier, New York: W. W. Norton, pp. 51–72.

Kraft, J. C., Kayan, I., & Erol, O. (1980), Geomorphic reconstructions in the environs of ancient Troy. *Science*, 209:776–782.

Larousse Encyclopedia of Mythology. New York: Prometheus Press, 1959.

Lattimore, R. (1951), *The Iliad of Homer.* Chicago: University of Chicago Press.

Lynd, H. M. (1958), *Shame and the Search of Identity.* New York: Harcourt Brace.

MacCary, W. T. (1982), *Childlike Achilles: Ontogeny and Phylogeny.* New York: Columbia University Press.

McCarthy, J. B. (1978), Narcissism and the self in homicidal adolescents. *Amer. J. Psychoanal.*, 38:19–29.

Marohn, R. C. (1991), Rage without content. Paper presented at the 14th Annual Conference on the Psychology of the Self. October 12, Chicago.

Morrison, A. P. (1983), Shame, the ideal self, and narcissism. *Contemp. Psychoanal.*, 19:295–318.

Nagy, G. (1979), *The Best of the Achaeans.* Baltimore: Johns Hopkins University Press.

—————— (1990), *Greek Mythology and Poetics.* Ithaca, NY: Cornell University Press.

North, H. (1966), *Saphrosyne, Self Knowledge and Self-Restraint in Greek Literature.* Ithaca, NY: Cornell University Press.

Parry, A. M. (1989), *The Language of Achilles and Other Papers.* Oxford: Clarendon Press.

Parry, M. (1971), *The Making of Homeric Verse: The Collected Papers of Milman Parry*, ed. A. Parry. Oxford: Oxford University Press.

Parson, E. R. (1984), The reparation of the self: Clinical and theoretical dimensions in the treatment of Vietnam combat veterans. *J. Contemp. Psychother.*, 14:4–56.

Piers, G., & Singer, M. B. (1971), *Shame and Guilt.* New York: W. W. Norton.

Redfield, J. M. (1975), *Nature and Culture in* The Iliad: *The Tragedy of Hector.* Chicago: University of Chicago Press.

Robertiello, R. C. (1976), Narcissism vs. instinct and object-love. *J. Contemp. Psychother.*, 8:11–14.

Rohde, E. (1898), *Psyche, Seelen Cult, und Unsterblichkeiteslaube der Greichen.* 9/10, Aufl. mit Einfuhrung von O. v. Weinreich. Tubingen, Ger: J. C. Mohr, 1925.

Rudolph, J. (1981), Aggression in the service of the ego and the self. *J. Amer. Psychoanal. Assn.*, 29:559–579.

Schein, S. L. (1984), *The Mortal Hero.* Berkeley: University of California Press.

Schore, A. N. (1991), Early superego development: The emergence of shame and narcissistic affect regulation in the practicing period. *Psychoanal. & Contemp. Thought*, 14:187–250.

—— (1992), A developmental psychoanalytic model of shame and narcissistic affect regulation. Paper presented to the Colloquium on Psychoanalysis and Affect: Early Object Relations, American College of Psychoanalysts. May.

Segal, C. (1971), *The Theme of Mutilation of the Corpse in the* Iliad. Leiden, Netherlands: E. J. Brill.

Shannon, R. S., III (1975), *The Arms of Achilles and Homeric Composition Technique.* Leiden, Netherlands: E. J. Brill.

Simon, B. (1978), *Mind and Madness in Ancient Greece.* Ithaca, NY: Cornell University Press.

Sinaiko, H. (1981), A study of the *Iliad.* Paper presented at the Chicago Society for Adolescent Psychiatry Winter Meeting, Lake Geneva, WI. February.

—— (1998), *Reclaiming the Canon.* New Haven, CT: Yale University Press.

Slater, P. E. (1968), *The Glory of Hera.* Boston: Beacon Press.

Snell, B. (1905), *The Discovery of the Mind,* tr. T. G. Rosenmeyer. New York: Dover Press, 1982.

Terman, D. M. (1975), Aggression and narcissistic rage: A clinical elaboration. *The Annual of Psychoanalysis*, 3:239–255. New York: International Universities Press.

Van Brock, N. (1959), Substitution rituelle. *Rev. Hittite et Asianique*, 65:117–146.

Weil, S. (1977), *The Iliad,* poem of might. *The Simone Weil Reader,* ed. G. A. Panichas. New York: David McKay, pp. 153–183.

Whitman, C. H. (1958), *Homer and the Homeric Tradition.* Cambridge, MA: Harvard University Press.

Wolf, E. S. (1988), *Treating the Self.* New York: Guilford Press.

Wood, E. (1985), *In Search of the Trojan War.* New York: Facts on File.

Yorke, C., with T. Balogh, P. Cohen, J. Davids, A. Gavshon, M. McCutcheon, J. D. McLean, J. Miller, & J. Szydlo (1990), The development and functioning of the sense of shame. *The Psychoanalytic Study of the Child.* 45:377–409. New Haven, CT: Yale University Press.

Chapter 8

Creativity in the Young Adult: A Partial Review and a Critique

And as imagination bodies forth
The forms of things unknown, the poet's pen
Turns them to shapes, and gives to airy nothing
A local habitation and a name
[Shakespeare, *A Midsummer's Night's Dream* 5. 1.
15–18].

This chapter will delineate at least two among many factors
that are important in the emergence of special creativity in
young adulthood (Sternberg and Davidson, 1983; Tannenbaum, 1986; Ostwald and Zegans, 1993). These factors are a
developmental readiness in terms of a process of consolidation
of an evolving personality and the construction of a special,
internalized object relationship combined with a highly invested interpersonal relationship between the artist and a significant person (Snyder, Benson, and Tessman, 1965; Rose,
1984). Smith and Carlsson have defined creativity as "a genera-
tive or productive way of experiencing reality, including the
perceiver's own self" (1990, p. 5). Currently creativity seems
to be studied via the delineation of various phenomena rather
than making a definitive discovery of the origins of creativity
(Stein and Heinze, 1960, cited by J. W. Anderson, 1980, p.
266). One of the problems with these definitions is that there

are so many different kinds of creativity; and there is more than one single characteristic that distinguishes talented people. In fact, Gardner and Wolf (1988) spell out five characteristics: neurobiological giftedness in artists occurs in the form of genetic and constitutional givens; special cognitive capacities, such as Freud's logical and linguistic skills and Picasso's visual–spatial skills; intense emotionality and ambition coupled with a high degree of self-confidence; an attraction to and a felicitous fitting in with a special intellectual domain; and the internal field of investigating the psychology of unconscious motivations. They suggest a combination of some or all these factors (though not necessarily with much synchrony), occurring in creative persons in some new way in the historical development of a scientific or artistic field. Gifted persons process information more quickly than the average; they construct rules and strategies to solve problems earlier and quicker; and make use of global strategies unknown to average people. The gifted person is challenged, stimulated, and motivated to solve problems others have stumbled over; for example, Newton's return mail solution of a problem the Bernouli brothers had struggled with for over a year. It could be said the creator achieves a kind of mastery of conflict between certain dualities and a "restoration of inner unity toward which we steadily strain" (Brenman-Gibson, 1976, p. 339). Brenman-Gibson sees man as a "playful" problem-finding, problem-making and problem-solving animal who sets up "contests" that increase in intensity and complexity with his moral and verbal development and appreciation of the sophisticated intricacies of interpersonal and intrapersonal experience. The artist, too, needs a "confirming response *from some audience*" (p. 349).

In line with the thesis presented here are some brief notes on creativity: William James at age 36 in 1878 began writing his *Principles of Psychology* (1890), on his honeymoon with Alice Howe Gibbens whose "admiration and support enabled him to confront and experiment with new ideas, and through her mirroring responses he was able to construct a more-reliable and better-individuated self-structure" (J. W. Anderson, 1980, p. 274) and "he read aloud every essay and every chapter of each book . . ." (p. 275); Virginia Woolf's husband Leonard was her principal support "becoming both a nursing companion and an acolyte of her divine madness, as he tolerantly perceived her mood disorder and shifting ego states . . ." (Abse, 1994, p. 23). Freud had his wife Martha, his friends Joseph Breuer, Wilhelm Fleiss, and later on his daughter Anna.

Joseph Conrad became a writer of fiction after he had abandoned his life on the sea and particularly so after his marriage to Jessie. His passive–dependent relationship with her, and his idealized, imagined close relationship with his uncle Thaddeus, and the later most significant relationship with his friend (and "secret sharer") Ford Madox Hueffer, provided the narcissistic supportive supplies he craved to free up his creativity that he used to work his way through various identity crises, a midlife crisis, fetishistic and oral fixations, depersonalization, and derealization (Joseph, 1963; Armstrong, 1971; Hamilton, 1975, 1979; Meyer, 1964a,b,c,d) that resulted from multiple traumatic losses: the loss of both parents, and his cousin Josephina, as well as a life-long struggle to maintain a cohesive personality. His creative writings, on the other hand, transcend his obvious neurotic conflicts. His skills of introspective exploration greatly assisted him in probing the depths of his characters' personalities to make them authentic and believable. Rising's study (1994) of *The Lagoon* lends a Kohutian interpretation, while the richness of Conrad's symbolic imagination, particularly in his greatest work, *The Heart of Darkness,* is creatively viewed from a classical psychoanalytic perspective by Sterba (1965) that enhances the appreciation of the story without detracting from the exquisite descriptive literature that draws the reader into Conrad's world of verdant and mortifying perceptions of the African landscape and the exploitation of the people there. Hamilton (1979) also describes the extraordinary deeply empathic "doppelganger" or fusion, communion relationship Conrad had with Bertrand Russell. After 1910 and his psychotic episode, Conrad's fiction became "stereotypical," his plots less "complex," and his characters more "alloplastic" (p. 178).

Even though the greatest American cubist and abstract painter, Manierre Dawson, was productive throughout his life, his most creative cubist and abstract work was done in his early twenties after he had married the beautiful Lili Boucher.

The study of the lives of famous creative individuals such as Beatrix Potter (Lane, 1946; Taylor, 1986, 1987; Hobbs, Whalley, and Taylor, 1987; Grinstein, 1995), Wordsworth (J. Wordsworth, 1987; Jeffrey, 1989), Strindberg (Lidz, 1964), and Coleridge (Mahon, 1987) has been quite popular, but brief vignettes like the ones cited above, as Ostwald and Zegans (1993) so clearly point out, without a depth psychological approach, with the exception of Grinstein's (1995) psychoanalytically informed study of Beatrix Potter, biographical data are interesting but are not necessarily explanatory enough for the discriminating reader (Greenacre, 1971; Spitz, 1985; J. Gedo, 1994; Meissner, 1994). Therefore, biographical data must be considered in a comprehensive examination of cognitive, conscious, preconscious, and unconscious aspects of creative individuals' motivations, imagination, and fantasy life.

Some researchers consider that postformal operations are critically necessary for creativity (Commons, Richards, and Armon, 1984). On the other hand, Koestler (1964, pp. 171–172) quotes Einstein's self-report of his intuitive, visual thinking that he considered most important. Keynes (1956) said the same about Newton's intuition in the solution of mathematical problems and physical phenomena. Einstein's genius (Miller, 1989), in fact, developed in the German intellectual milieu of a visual mode of mental imagery, intuition, and abstractions from observable facts. He had studied algebra and geometry since the age of 8 with the encouragement of his uncle Jakob who was very sophisticated in mathematics. Jakob challenged his nephew with complicated math problems, and this stimulus was critically important in his nephew's development since Einstein worked on these problems for many hours in solitude, thus perfecting his logical *and* intuitive skills. This was followed later on with his experiments regarding the theory of light and the relative speed of falling objects. Einstein tried to put himself in tune with the Creator of a marvelously complex, intricate, and interconnected universe (Lubin, 1977). Whether creativity emanates from illusions (Gombrich, 1961; Gomrich, Hochberg, and Black, 1970), fantasies, postformal operations, visual imaginings, or a primitive "oceanic" feeling state (Koestler, 1964), one must most of all be modest, like Freud (1908) in approaching this complicated subject. The concepts here are in keeping with that injunction.

These two factors (consolidation of the personality and an intense relationship with another person), I repeat, are *not the only ones* present in special creativity, and this contribution is neither an exhaustive analysis of the subject nor a complete review of the voluminous literature, since many attempts to understand *the key* (Hershman and Lieb, 1988) to this problem at any age have opened up many complex, contradictory, and controversial observations and speculations (Koestler, 1964; Fossi, 1985; J. E. Gedo, 1988; Boorstin, 1992; Palombo, 1992). Besides, there are many different kinds of creativity.

Musical and mathematical creativity are often matched together, but linguistic and empathic skills are rarely connected to interests in mathematics or physics. Also, there is the exposure of the myth of single authorship in the well-known collaboration of such artists as Picasso with Bracque (M. Gedo, 1980) and Van Gogh with Gaugin (Brettell, Cachin, Freches-Thory, and Stuckey 1988), as well as the early Impressionists with each other (Tinterow and Loyrette, 1994); Wordsworth both with Coleridge, and a host of Wordsworth's relatives; Coleridge's extensive verbatim "borrowings" from the German philosophers; Ezra Pound's editing of T. S. Eliot's poetry; J. S. Mill with Harriet Taylor Mill (1970); Keats with his editors; both Thomas Wolfe and F. Scott Fitzgerald were heavily edited by Maxwell Perkins; and Faulkner collaborated extensively with his editor Saxe Commins (Stillinger, 1991). Piaget and Inhelder (1967), Feldman (1971, 1974), and Walters and Gardner (1986) have described these collaborations, but Gardner's concept is one of certain "crystallizing" experiences arising from "powerful catalytic forces" (Gardner, 1982 p. 42) that are irreversible. In fact, Feldman (1991) states that Mozart's older sister Nannerl's musical performances on the piano facilitated or "crystallized" the development of Mozart's genius. New and exciting musical knowledge was assimilated into an existing native structure of extraordinary musical ability. Expanding on Piaget's notion of a mixture of "unique intellectual, emotional, social, and spiritual qualities in an individual" (p. 36, 1982), whose giftedness necessarily depends on a rich environment to germinate and evolve. In summary Feldman (1982) believes that extraordinary mastery of a field is the result of a prolonged, systematic, and guided interaction with specific environmental forces such as teachers, peers, educational materials, technologies, competitions, and performances: (see also Feldman, 1971, 1974, 1982, 1986, 1991).

These crystallizing experiences are derived from universal sources in the evolutionarily derived human, certain cultural sources, and then creative building on another's contribution to a field. Crystallizing experiences involve exceptional talent in a person combined with unusual and remarkable contact with certain materials in the domain in which the talent is manifested. Young adults seem to have initiating crystallizing experiences while older persons have refining ones. This concept of a significant relationship germinating, facilitating, and crystallizing creativity is consistent with many psychoanalysts' experiences of observing patients with potential talent, then creativity emerges late in their analyses following the working through of neurotic conflicts. For example, one young adult professional man long interested in creative writing but neurotically unable to use these skills, began to write emotionally laden poetry toward the end of a very successful analysis. Another man developed a remarkable ability to integrate and synthesize extremely complex abstract theories during the later phase of his analysis.

THEORETICAL CONSIDERATIONS

The terms *creativity, giftedness,* or *talent* and *genius* are often used interchangeably, and to avoid confusion Feldman (1982) has offered a useful classification: giftedness "refers to the achievement of advanced levels of mastery in a specified domain—for example, a successful concert pianist. . . . Creativity goes beyond this level to include adding a new meaning to the existing domain: a concert pianist's interpretation of a Mozart sonata that finds new, fresh meaning. . . ." Genius refers to a total "reorganization of an entire domain" (p. 41), for example, Freud's development of psychoanalysis, Einstein's contributions regarding the physical properties of gravity, relativity, and light, and Darwin's contributions to biology and evolutionary theory. A satisfactory commonsense definition is Jacques Barzun's (1989) summary: "from productivity in the work place, to ordinary artistic endeavors for one's own use, to commercial and professional art forms and finally to the highest level of genius" (p. 343). For the sake of clarity, however, creativity is used here in the broader sense including all three categories. Gardner's uniquely helpful list of special talents (1982) are:

"[A]utonomous intellectual competencies": linguistic competence, such as that exhibited by writers and public speakers; musical competence, such as that found in composers and performers; mathematical–logical competence, or the kinds of problem-solving abilities studied by Piaget and realized to a high degree by scientists; visual–spatial competence, such as the ability to envision and transform visual–spatial representations found in artists, [architects and engineers]; bodily–kinesthetic competence, such as the abilities exploited by athletes and dancers; social–interpersonal competence, or the abilities needed for successful interaction with other individuals, such as the skills found in politicians with groups [and psychoanalysts with individuals]; intrapersonal competence, or knowledge of and access to one's own feelings and desires; self knowledge [such as found in psychoanalysts] [Gardner, 1982, p. 52].

Jerome Bruner (1968) as quoted by Feldman (1974) "defines creativity as the occurrence of 'effective surprise' in an individual who has produced a work and/or someone who comprehends and appreciates that work for the first time" (p. 58). Once a discovery has been made it seems so obvious that we are surprised no one thought of it before, and it evokes wonderment and astonishment.

The creative person has a high tolerance for complexity; he protests and challenges current perceptions of reality; he has a heightened degree of introspection and a fluidity of boundaries between self and object similar to adolescent processes (Blos, 1962). According to Ernest Jones (1956) Freud maintained a mixture of skepticism and naiveté that allowed him to give free rein to new ideas and speculations that he matched up with a scientific approach.

Wherever and whenever creativity occurs it attracts our attention because the creator generates something excitingly novel, yet at the same time the product may be quite simple and the creator does so repeatedly. Creative individuals break new ground in science, literature, and art notably in the case of Leonardo da Vinci, Galileo, the Curies, Newton, Gauss, Einstein, Freud, Shakespeare, and Goethe, who come to mind in this regard since they all created new fields. The people we regard as geniuses have extraordinary capacities for perceiving reality in new ways, analogies and similarities amongst dissimilarities. They are blessed with a curious, questioning, wondering sensitivity and an especially perceptive, assimilative mind that is responsive to fresh stimuli that excite a multitude of different trains of thought. Polanyi (1969), Koestler (1964), Mednick (1962), and De Bono (1969) as cited by Noy (1985) all refer to the same process of the artist perceiving, challenging, rearranging, and recombining reality in revolutionary and different ways. They "wrench," as it were, a new perception out from conventional perceptions of reality. Noy (1985), using a computer analogy, suggests artists use a "habitual" cognitive style or a "prolific" repertoire of internalized programs for processing information. The artist or scientist, he says, experiments with new ways of solving problems that augment the "repertoire of programs in order to improve steadily their ability to solve problems" (p. 425). Noy (1985) further suggests an openness and readiness in artists and scientists to accept "irrational" or primary processlike thinking, and they openly court novelty that for him is "the most interesting ability of the creative individual" (p. 430). This "preconscious processing makes free use of analogy and allegory, superimposing dissimilar ingredients into new perceptual and conceptual patterns, thus reshuffling experience to achieve that extraordinary degree of condensation without which creativity in any field would be impossible" (Kubie, 1967, p. 38). Feldman (1986) and Weisberg and Springer (1961) add that the families of such individuals are consistently receptive and encouraging of this ability (e.g., the prolific Bach family), as well as there being an acceptance by a larger society that the creative artist early on perceives and most particularly anticipates the interests, trends, or needs of society. In fact, Noy (1985) suggests, too, that there is an active interrelationship "between the creative artist and the historical development of science and art" (p. 435). Koestler makes the same point about a "ripeness of a culture for a new synthesis since multiple discoveries are made around the same time" (p. 120), such as the independent work of Darwin and Wallace on natural selection as well as Newton and Liebnitz on calculus.

Similar to families with several creative individuals, the high frequency of outstanding work done in certain university academic departments is very striking and it is no small coincidence that more than any other department, six consecutive Nobel prizes (eight altogether: Papajohn, 1995) have been awarded in recent years to several members of the Economics Department at the University of Chicago. The suggestion here is that the toughening and healthily competitive intellectual sociopsychological environment in that department incubated, nurtured, facilitated, and fostered outstanding continuing creative work amongst its members. It seems imminently clear that genius rarely, if ever, occurs in isolation (Stillinger, 1991).

Another way of looking at the creative individual is Gruber's (1982, 1989) "evolving systems approach" wherein the development of giftedness in such persons as Darwin, Freud, and Piaget occurs over a lifetime of study and work within an evolving milieu. The case study method allows for the examination of each unique creative individual who "is a coherent knowing system" and whose work is "original," "purposeful," and "harmonious or compatible with other human purposes, needs and values" (Gruber, 1989, p. 4). The artist sets out to be creative and defines the working self in a network of related enterprises.

His ideas evolve over time in a series of smaller insights that build into larger insights.

The greatest psychologist before Freud in terms of introspection and self-exploration was Saint Augustine. His *Confessions* was the very first autobiography in history, and in the very first chapter, Augustine recalls details of his childhood development, the process of language development, and he accurately describes the processes of grief and mourning for a friend who died (p. 53). They were like each other's alter ego: "one soul in two bodies" (p. 54). But it was his relationship to God and his mother's relentless pursuit that was central to his religious conversion as well as his spiritual and creative development (Kligerman, 1957). Joyce's (1916) *A Portrait of the Artist* is a very interesting account of a young adult's struggles to grow up. Likewise Proust's (1981) monumental self-portrait is currently enjoying a literary revival. See also Richardson's autobiographical story (Richardson, 1989; Wallace, 1989).

Wordsworth's autobiographical *Prelude* (Reed, 1991) was written and rewritten over forty years, the subtitle of which is "The Growth of a Poet's Mind." It was originally addressed to Coleridge when Wordsworth and Dorothy were in Germany in 1798. Coleridge and Wordsworth were collaborators, but it was Wordsworth's one-year younger sister Dorothy who was more of an alter ego. She kept a journal that provided both her brother and Coleridge with raw material for poems, notably the poem "Daffodils," and was a source of constant interchange and support before and after his marriage to Mary Hutchinson and the birth of their children. Coleridge's frustrated and unrequited love for Mary's sister Sara is in fact thought to have been a major reason for his depressions and opium addiction. Linda Jeffrey's "Writing and Rewriting Poetry: William Wordsworth" (1989) illuminates the thesis that Wordsworth's creativity involved much repetition, revising, and reiterating. Not only is repetition a common poetic device, but it seems to be a central part of all creativity. In "Daffodils" (1804, 1815) reflection upon a scene viewed earlier is recaptured in vivid detail to create a wonderfully fresh perception.

Wordsworth, Coleridge, Keats, Blake, Shelley, Turner, and Constable similarly were especially moved by nature and became known as the innovators of the Romantic Movement in English literature and art (Pinsky, 1988). Wordsworth wrote the familiar poem about the rainbow and Constable painted several canvases of rainbows. Wordsworth's memories of his childhood, adolescence, and youth provided the stimulation and content of his poetry. Often he wrote the poems in notebooks from the back to the front and combined memory of past events with commentary about those memories. As in analysis, he used prolonged contemplation, recollection, reiteration, and revision as forms of thinking. He organized and structured his thoughts in this manner, and childhood memories were reworked and filtered through his adult personality. He said poetry was "emotion recollected in tranquility," but he also said poetry was "the science of emotion." In fact, the therapeutic effects of his poetry are attested to by none other than J. S. Mill who said he recovered from a period of depression while reading Wordsworth's poetry. Wordsworth's greatest period of creativity occurred in the decade between his twenty-seventh and thirty-seventh years (1797 to 1806), after he had recovered from a kind of mental breakdown or identity crisis (J. Wordsworth, 1987, p. 4; Reed, 1991, p. 38). Somewhat earlier (ages 21–22), he was so emotionally enthralled with the French Revolution, he traveled to France, met a young woman there, Annette Vallon, who bore him a daughter Caroline whom he supported, but the war between France and England prevented him from going back to marry Annette. This emotional crisis and the failure of the revolution was tremendously disillusioning. As a result, he had a major emotional crisis that in effect was a reliving of the traumatic loss of both parents at

8 (mother) and 11 (father). His said his feelings and faculties were generated and "quickened" by the relationship with his mother:

> Nurs'd in his mother's arms, the Babe who sleeps
> Upon his Mother's breast, who, when his soul
> Claims manifest kindred with an earthly soul
> Doth gather passion from his mother's eye!
> [Book II, 240–243].

Her death left him without "props." He meditated on the transience of life and the experience of loss and suffering that he "managed in terms of an interaction between the individual mind and Nature, . . . ([that] the German philosophers Ficte, Schelling and Hegel) called the self and the other, or subject and object" (see for example the poems *Tintern Abbey and Ode to Intimations of Immortality* [Abrams, 1987, p. ix; Pinsky, 1988]). Love of nature was transformed into the higher ideals of love for liberty and mankind and his "imaginative human mind, which is dependent for its creative freedom on love" (Reed, 1987, p. 38). His relationships with his sister Dorothy, his wife Mary, and later his friend Coleridge fostered this transformation. It is interesting to speculate that he was inspired by living in Milton's former rooms at Cambridge. Returning home for the summer after the first year at Cambridge, mourning the loss of his mother, he wept on his former landlady's grave like the Wolf Man who wept on Pushkin's grave as a substitute for sorrow at the death of his sister. When walking around the neighborhood lake and greeting his neighbors, Wordsworth restored and transmuted his sad "weariness" and was "wrapp'd and sooth'd" (Book IV, 153). He drank in the delights of nature:

> My body from the stillnes drinking in
> A restoration like the calm of sleep

But sweeter far. Above, before, behind,
Around me, All was peace and solitude:

[Book IV, 386–389].

He grieved the loss of his mother:

Early died
My honour'd Mother; she who was the heart
And hinge of all our learnings and our loves
She left us destitute, and as we might
Trooping together [Book V, 256–260].

In the same vein, Wordsworth recalls the death of a boy of
10 and a man who suicided by drowning in the lake. But then
he aspired to something loftier and turned to the ideal of hu-
mankind:

Lifted above the ground by airy fancies
More bright than madness or the dreams of wine
And, though full oft the objects of our love
Were false, and in their splendour overwrought,
Yet, surely, at such time no vulgar power
Was working in us, nothing less in truth
Than that most noble attribute of man,
Though yet untutor'd and inordinate
That wish for something loftier, more adorn'd
Than is the common aspect, daily garb
Of human life [Book V, 591–601].

Wordsworth then, like so many late adolescents and young
adults, after three winters at college (Cambridge) tired of academic life, blew off the exams, and traveled with a classmate
to the Alps, that had the effect of solidifying an evolving personality in the process.

Melville (Tolchin, 1988) specifically processed in his novels
the way his various characters dealt with grief that mirrored his
mourning the loss of his father at age 12. His mother's strong

influence led to his identifying with her so-called feminized Victorian style of suppressing all feelings about loss. Tolchin's implicit and explicit assumption here is that Melville's creativity arose from this unfinished and delayed mourning process. This concept of delayed grief and mourning certainly influenced the content of Melville's writings, but his creativeness stemmed from his special gift not just in mastery of the mourning process, since after *Moby Dick* his talent was overcome by the very same unfinished grief and his inherited manic–depressive tendencies. One could argue just the opposite, that his mother's stoic resolve held the family together just enough and provided sufficient strength that opposed whatever corrosion of controls were deployed against the overwhelming traumatic memories of his father's horrible and feverish railings at his death. With these caveats in mind, the manner in which Tolchin cites the personalities of the characters in the novels and constructs his thesis, is very intriguing and interesting, if not convincing, for the main thesis that Melville's creativity arose from the uncompleted mourning.

Keegan (1989) traces Darwin's development as a geological scientist first and secondarily how he became interested in biology, and later still in mind and emotion when his son was born. His knowledge of geology helped him develop his theory of gradualism for both the individual of a species and the group composed of individuals. He considered that physical and mental traits evolve over time to benefit both the individual and the group. Keegan asserts that Darwin's creative thinking emerged from one area of expertise to another. Darwin's contact with John Gould, the most prominent ornithologist of the day, made him a confirmed evolutionist in 1836. This seems to have been true also for Edelman who won a Nobel prize for his work on the immune system before entering neuroscience where he has made and continues to make additional significant discoveries.

Does genius really begin in adolescence? Blos (1962), H. H. Anderson (1965), and J. W. Anderson (1980) seem to think so. Eissler (1978) cites the case of the adolescent Freud whose love for Gisela Fluss was thwarted and served as a traumatic motivation for a sturdy set of delaying defenses against libidinal desires that postponed the onset of his creative endeavors. The same could be said for Mozart whose early childhood and adolescent libidinal development was guided, controlled, suppressed, and delayed by his father Leopold so that he was totally immersed in music as the darling prodigy of royalty (Solomon, 1995). Adolescence is developmentally full of many changes, and creativity is commonly and closely associated with change, since the creator perceives the need for changing the way reality is received and represented. The creative person is involved in a developmental readiness for exercising his talent.

The creative person is like an adolescent or young adult who courageously and fearlessly confronts convention in the universe of the sciences or the arts and often is so focused (Rathunde and Csikszentmihalyi, 1993) from within that he is willing to suffer bitter poverty or other forms of deprivation in order to pursue invention (Van Gogh, Monet, Vivaldi, and Bartok come to mind). Handel, for example, while composing the *Messiah*, confined himself to his rooms for three weeks, frequently forgetting to eat. Likewise, Mozart, while under pressure to compose, didn't take time to eat or sleep. He constantly drummed his fingers and was engrossed in an internal musical activity (Ostwald, 1993; Ostwald and Zegans, 1993, p. 172). Creative persons seem to be blessed with a remarkable characteristic of being oblivious to the passage of time (Eissler, 1971, p. 27). In fact, creative persons possess an unusual capacity for prolonged and "sustained attention" (W. James, 1890, p. 423); "their ideas coruscate, every subject branches infinitely before their fertile minds, and for hours they remain rapt" (p. 423). A perfect example is when Gauss arrived at new mathematical constructions after days and weeks of concentrated thought. It was as though he couldn't rest until he had found a solution to a problem. John Maynard Keynes (1956) said the same about Newton whose "peculiar gift was the power of holding continuously in his mind a purely mental problem until he had seen straight through it [and] surrendered to him its secret" (p. 278). Keynes added that "his pre-eminence is due to his muscles of intuition being the strongest and most enduring with which man has ever been gifted" (p. 278). Newton, "the archetype of the experimental, empirical scientist" (Westfall, 1981, p. 342) was similar to Gauss in this respect, except Newton readily provided immediate answers to problems. Besides, Newton was blessed with "being a supreme mathematical technician, he could dress it up, how you will, for purposes of exposition, but it was his intuition which was pre-eminently extraordinary—'so happy in his conjectures,' said de Morgan as to seem to know more than he could possibly have any means of proving" (Newman, 1956, p. 278). In fact, Newton frequently came up with mathematical proofs in a flash of brilliance. However, as a sort of social isolate Newton's creative contributions to science were not directly related to the crystallizing relationship with a special person, even though he was very close to his mother. His life is a significant contradiction to one part of the thesis presented here, but does conform to the other important factor: namely, a major consolidation and synthesis of creative elements in an early young adulthood personality.

What role does imagination play? Gifted persons certainly have a fertile and playful imagination that is part of the development of their talents (Panel, 1959; Kohut, 1959; Greenacre, 1959). Coleridge's capacity for symbolism in his imagination is very evident in his poetry, especially *The Rime of the Ancient Mariner* (Mahon, 1987) and *Kubla Khan* (Barth, 1977). Coleridge differentiated imagination from fantasy (fancy). He idolized Wordsworth's many virtues, preeminent of which was his imagination that led to a creative synthesis of "opposite or discordant qualities"; "idea and image; the individual and the representative; novelty and familiarity; emotions and order; judgement and feeling; the natural and the artificial; the poet and the poem" (Barth, 1977, p. 49). Imagination, he claimed, is the "soul" of the poet's genius.

A psychoanalytic structural perspective can be understood as the presence of a relatively "porous" repression barrier. Anna Freud (1981), in fact, claimed creative artists have a greater capacity for insight since the usual barriers between the conscious and unconscious regions are more porous, though not necessarily weak, and that makes for receptivity to primary process imagery and availability to consciousness of ideas and feelings. Similarly, Leavey (1970) inferred the same thing in John Keats' capacity to give free rein to his imagination. Kohut's consideration of this situation was that the "psychic organization of some creative people is characterized by a fluidity of the basic narcissistic configuration of the personality . . ." (1966, p. 189), that allows them to regressively gain access to the creative elements in the unconscious and then with the help of certain special cognitive structures pull together the disparate elements into something novel. These cognitive structures are categorization, abstraction, context, and association (Noy, 1978).

The creative mind escapes the "straitjacket imposed on it by the inflexible categorization modes of intellect and language and to create new and original categories" (Noy, 1978, p. 721). Formal operations of abstraction are converted into visual or auditory stimuli. The creative person freely shifts from one context of particular elements to another and then reorganizes those elements. Associational patterns shift from logical to illogical. These same factors are observed clinically in the best of analytic patients as they acquire insight and learn to make creative use of free association to ferret out unconscious meanings to interpret their own dreams and become familiar with structured unconscious fantasies and personal myths.

Margaret Brenman-Gibson has written extensively on creativity and in a similar vein:

> It is man's nature, by way of his *visionary propensity*, to try in a multitude of forms to resolve dualities and to dissolve boundaries, in order to restore a measure of that harmonious earliest reality (with its sense of unified wholeness and centrality), which we can presume was all-encompassing in the warm waters of the womb and thereafter re-experienced in the relation of the nursing infant to mother as he looks at her face beaming down upon him. This boundary-less unity is perhaps the prototype of feeling "at home with everything" and in harmony with the universe [1976, p. 337].

Amy Lowell said the creative artist is "a man of extraordinarily sensitive and active subconscious personality, fed by, and feeding a nonresistant consciousness" (Ghiselin, 1952, p. 110). She differs, like Kris (1952), from Freud in claiming the psychic state of creativity is "not a daydream, but an entirely different psychic state and one peculiar to itself" (p. 110).[1] While she may be right that creative efforts are not just daydreams, Freud (1907, 1908) drew some very important similarities between creative writing and daydreaming (see, Person, Fonagy, and Figueira, 1995).

Some researchers have likened this state to a sort of trance filled with emotional feelings from the depths of the unconscious that is in turn subjected to an organizing, cognitive structuralizing influence. An often quoted example is Kekule's

---

[1]Repetition is also a very real part of learning and the laying down of memory. Jeffrey (1989) points out that practicing is an important element of Piaget's theory of the development of mind from the repeating of the mind's capacity to reflect and extract the emotional essence of childhood memories. These schemata are similar to Mahler's developmental practicing subphase of separation-individuation and the process in analysis of working through.

famous description of his discovery of the benzene ring (Japp, 1898, p. 100) during a half-conscious reverie while watching the leaping flames in the fireplace that suggested a snake grasping its tail in its mouth (Kekule, 1865, quoted in Findlay, 1937).

> I was sitting, writing at my textbook; but the work did not progress; my thoughts went elsewhere. I turned my chair to the fire and dozed. Again the atoms were gamboling before my eyes. This time the smaller groups kept modestly in the background. My mental eye, rendered more acute by repeated visions of the kind, could now distinguish larger structures, of manifold conformation: long rows, sometimes more closely fitted together; all twining and twisting in snake-like motion, but look! What was that? one of the snakes had seized hold of its own tail, and the form whirled mockingly before my eyes. As if by a flash of lightening I awoke; and this time also I spent the rest of the night working out the consequences of the hypothesis [quoted in Findlay, 1937, p. 43].

That was in 1865, but eleven years earlier, he was in a similar state of reverie while riding a London bus. He visualized the carbon and hydrogen atoms "gamboling" to form a chain. He then put to paper his formulae of organic chemical chains. Obviously, he had been thinking long and hard about how to visualize organic compounds and thus he ushered in a revolution in that field. The fact he had trained as a architect also was especially helpful in his visual imagination. Secondary reworking of the erroneously termed "sudden" inspiration of the skeletal outlines of an idea was characteristic alike of Wordsworth, the poet, and Poincaré, the mathematician. Most creative people report that creative activity merely appears to be sudden or easy. Indeed, much effort and thought is often involved in revising and reworking of a piece several times over that is not at all unusual. For example, Leonardo reworked his painting of Mona Lisa for many years right up until his death, and Beethoven repeatedly revised the last movements of his

Hammerklavier Sonata and *Fifth Symphony*. Tchaikovsky worked on his extraordinary *Romeo and Juliet Fantasy Overture* for ten years (Huscher, 1995). Brahms reworked his *First Symphony* over many years. Wordsworth's working papers reveal the same incessant revising process.

Koestler (1964) proposes a "bisociation" process of mental operations taking place on two different planes or "matrices." For example, Gutenberg's invention of the printing press came from his observations of the manufacture of playing cards by transferring onto paper the images from wood blocks and then observing the wine press squeeze out the grape juice in the production of wine. The idea struck him that type could be made from the soft metal, lead, that when inked could be pressed onto paper (Koestler, 1964, pp. 122–123).

From a structural point of view, Kris's concept of regression in the service of the ego (1952) in the development of the creative process does not necessarily involve a pathological change in personality or self organization since it describes in ego psychological language the stages of inspiration and elaboration. Kubie (1958) locates creative activity in the preconscious where certain orientations, connections, and observations are imprinted. Arnheim (1976) adds the concept of visual symbolic thinking that resides in the preconscious. Pinchas Noy (1968, 1969, 1978, 1979, 1985) has extended this concept further with a feedback kind of interplay between the primary and secondary processes that results in new structure formation in the "upper" layer(s) of the otherwise so-called inchoate cauldron of primary process functioning. At any rate, it is from this area of the personality that creativity is thought to be derived. Liebert (1983) has put it rather succinctly:

> The work of art is actually the outgrowth of a continuously cycling biphasic process which involves, at first, a regression to more primitive primary process modes of thought (the inspiration phase) and then the ideas are subjected to the synthetic

capacity to transform the dim awareness of the turbulent interior into a form that has the redeeming value of appearing real
in itself as well as both communicative and pleasurable to the
beholder [p. 7].

Nass (1984) disagrees with Kris's formulation. Specifically,
he refutes the notion of regression (though he doesn't differentiate nonpathological from pathological phenomena), since
the capacity to employ ambiguous affective and cognitive states
implies ego strength and "builds upon the . . . capacity to
maintain contact with early body and self states" (p. 485). He
interviewed twenty musical composers and learned that gestures and body rhythms of kinesthetic experience (related to
Piaget's sensorimotor concepts and Schilder's linking motility
to perception) play a role in musical composition. These perceptions include visual, tactile, kinesthetic, as well as auditory
sensations that tap into early childhood separation experiences. Polanyi also refutes the notion of regression and proposes a subsidiary awareness that is neither preconscious nor
unconscious but is instead a functional degree of conscious
"foreknowledge of what we call a problem" (1969, p. 60) that
calls for a solution. Polanyi also calls for a two-step process: a
deliberate focal act of imagination is followed by a "spontane-
ous coordination of visual cues" (pp. 64–65). "The imagination sallies forward, and intuition integrates what the
imagination has lit upon" (Polanyi, 1969, p. 64).

Rothenberg (1990) has described another two-stage process
that is most innovative and novel, the first of which he calls
the "janusian process." He arrived at his ideas from many nonclinical interviews with modern creative poets and novelists.
This rather novel idea of "nonconscious" cognition purports
that the artist or scientist conceives of "multiple opposites or
antitheses that are conceived simultaneously, either as existing

side by side or as equally operative, valid, or true ... the creative person consciously formulates the simultaneous operation of antithetical elements or factors and develops those formulations into integrated entities or creations" (p. 15). Logic is defied or ignored. The second stage is the "homospatial process" whereby two disparate ideas or perceptions occur "fleetingly" side by side or superimposed on each other and then fuse followed by a new integration that emerges out of this fusion.

Truly, creativity, as Ghiselin (1952) points out, is a "process of change, of development, of evolution, in the organization of subjective life" (p. 12) and it "begins typically with a vague, even a confused excitement, some sort of yearning, a hunch, or some other preverbal intimation of approaching or potential resolution ... preceded by a muddled suspense" (p. 14). The motivation is part of an inborn curiosity or exploratory drivenness to find novelty. The choice of subject matter is very selective and not just random for the creative person whether poet, mathematician, or composer, since an inner pressured voice is listened to in the creative act. Writers (notably Virginia Woolf) often say they have to write, something that Greenacre (1971) referred to as the artist's need to create, and likened the act of creation to a "love affair with the world" or as she called it a "libidinization" of the piece and the creator offers his "love gift" (p. 490) to an imaginary collective audience that he believes will be greatly appreciative.

Greenacre (1971) wrote about the exquisite sensitiveness to the external world in the first year of life in gifted persons. This sensitivity is initially mastered by creating what she called "collective alternates," a term similar to Winnicott's concepts (1951) of transitional objects and transitional shared space. The gifted infant responds, Greenacre claims, with particular creative sensitiveness to the multiple sensory experiences of

the feeding situation including olfactory, visual, auditory, proprioceptive, temperature, touch, the rhythms, and forms of
maternal behaviors. More importantly, what should be added
to this list is the empathic exchange between mother and infant. This sensitivity is especially retained and refined,
Greenacre says, throughout the artist's development.

> Thus we can conceive of the fact that for the potentially gifted
> infant the primary object which stimulates certain sensory re-
> sponses to it is invested with a greater field of related experi-
> ences than would not be true for the less gifted infant of lesser
> endowment. As part of this reaction, too, there would inevitably
> be a greater vibration and need for harmonizing the inner ob-
> ject relationships . . . (pp. 489–490).

In a way, Greenacre is anticipating here some of Kohut's
theory of development of the bipolar self through multiple
interactions with selfobjects. Kohut (1966), however, considers
creativity as one of the transformations of narcissism. He refers
to an idealization of a piece of work that is experienced as part
of the self and cites as evidence that artists invest their work
with narcissistic libido, particularly when they vacillate between
cycles of overvaluing and undervaluing their productions. Furthermore, he believes that the artist is more childlike in his
wide-eyed, fresh approach to perceiving novelty in the midst
of commonality as well as being "less psychologically separated
from his surroundings . . . i.e., the You–I barrier is not clearly
defined" (p. 112). Also, Kohut (1976) was the first to postulate
a "transference of creativity" whereby the creative person es-
tablishes a transference with a significant other person during
the work of creation, such as Freud's relationship with Wilhelm
Fleiss during his self-analysis, that led to Freud's great achievement of creating the science and art of psychoanalysis. This
"transference of creativity" is similar to the archaic transferences that occur in the analysis of certain narcissistic personalities. Kohut said that during periods of intense creative activity

the self is enfeebled by a withdrawal of investments in the self to concentrate on the creative task.

Abse (1994), in discussing John Keats, refers to a similar process of "absorption of the poet in the creative process, which resulted in his work often reflecting deletion of self-consciousness and fusion of the subject (the poet) and his subject matter (his object world)" (p. 28). The most common transference of creativity is an idealizing one where the artist or scientist feels depleted in the creative effort and needs to obtain strength from an idealizing object. Another form of transference of creativity is like the mirror transference where the need is to be confirmed by an admiring other.

Elisabeth Young-Bruehl (1991) has described what she calls the character ideal occurring in several forms of character development. Similar to the thesis presented in this chapter, she feels that this function derives from a consolidated personality in late adolescence, but she goes on to indicate that it is the internal structure "character ideal" that is responsible for creativity. What is open to question here is whether there is such an architectonic or even a psychological structure of a character ideal, or is it rather a dynamically fluid motivating influence that is responsible for the creative process? What seems lacking in Young-Bruehl's theory is her emphasis solely on a cognitive structure without a consideration of global external and internal influences including a special emphasis on an active (internal or external) relationship with a significant person.

From all the foregoing research in the field of creativity it is clear the status of research is in an early stage of observing and recording of the phenomena. No definitive overarching theory has yet emerged amongst the various contributions. From whatever theoretical framework one approaches this subject of creativity, it seems especially important to note that creative individuals are uniquely and sensitively receptive. Furthermore, they are gifted with special cognitive functions of perceptual sensitivities and visual–spatial skills that make them freely available to respond to the rudimentary seminal ideas arising from an inspiration in the unconscious. Leonardo da Vinci had this remarkable capacity to combine creative thinking and painterly action in a way more novel than his nearest competitor. In line with the thesis in this chapter, Wallace and Gruber (1989) and Stein and Heinze (1960) have proposed the study of individual cases to illustrate some intrinsic issues in creativity.

Erikson's approach includes developmental and psychosocial points of view and he emphasizes the psychobiographical aspects of his subjects' lives such as his studies of Luther (1958) and Gandhi (1969) while Muslin's and Jobe's self psychological approach to the study of Lyndon Johnson (1991) and Muslin's work on Hitler and Gandhi (1995) is a new way of addressing this complicated subject. Yet another and incomparable model is Liebert's (1983) monumental study of Michelangelo whose thorough treatment of the man, his work, and his intense and ambivalent relationship with Pope Julius bring the artist to life without reductionistic minimizing. Both Ernest Jones's (1953, 1955, 1957) and Peter Gay's (1988) biographies of Freud each in their own way provide us with much data that construct a fuller understanding of Freud's genius and document the intense transference–countertransference relationship he had with Fliess that was especially important in Freud's development of his creative contributions.

The life summarized here is that of the Victorian moralist (Himmelfarb, 1994) and novelist George Eliot[2] who "emerged" on the literary scene on February 4, 1857, at the age of 37. This identity, which meant *ELIOT—To Lewes I Owe It*, was as humorously designed as the private names she and George

---

[2]The inspiration for some of the ideas in this chapter comes from Ruby Redinger's magnificent biography of George Eliot (1975).

Henry Lewes used for each other: "Mother" and "Madonna" (G. E. Eliot was "Madonna"). Their home was jokingly called "The Priory." She derived George from Lewes and also Georges Sand, whom she greatly admired and identified with. She was similar to Georges Sand in that she apparently had a strong sexual interest, except in Eliot it was focused exclusively on men. Women writers of literary ambition in the Victorian era, it must be remembered, were usually obliged to hide their identities, although Charlotte Bronte was courageous enough not to hide hers.

George Eliot was baptized Mary Anne Evans in 1819, the youngest of three children born in a second marriage to a moderately successful land agent. From 1850 to 1880 she signed all her personal correspondence as Marian. In 1880, she reverted to Mary Ann, having dropped the "e" from Anne earlier. For the time she lived with Lewes she was Marian or Mrs. George Henry Lewes. After Lewes died, she married a family friend, John W. Cross, twenty years her junior, because she was very needy and could not bear to live alone. Her identity was rather fluid and not fully formed until she began her relationship with Lewes. Redinger (1975) makes the cardinal point that Eliot did not emerge as a literary genius until she had settled into her relationship with Lewes. Until that time her personality was submerged, incomplete, and "arrested" from living in a rigid and repressive atmosphere. Furthermore, she didn't have the courage or enough internal cohesion to break away from her past until her relationship with Lewes had flowered two whole years after they had met. Redinger (1975) carefully documented the process of Eliot's separation and individuation as a person and as a writer. It is an authentic account of a naturally occurring evolution that reminds one of a successful psychoanalytic therapeutic experience. The following is a summary of her life experience along with a psychoanalytic interpretation of her development into young adulthood and her emergence as a major author.

Her first attachment, of course, was to her mother, but her mother was rarely mentioned in her letters except to acknowledge the fact that everyone has a mother. The obvious conclusion is that this primary attachment was not all that strong or lasting to begin with. Moreover, the mother was sickly, especially following George Eliot's birth, and at 2 years of age George Eliot was deposited in the Victorian version of a day-care center, and at 6 years she was sent away to a boarding school like her two older siblings. As a small child, she was very attached to her older brother Isaac, tagging along after him in all his activities. Her mother thought she was too much of a tomboy and she never really had a normal childhood. Eliot had idolized Isaac, and reminiscing at 25, she wrote some idyllic verse (her Sonnets) about their childhood relationship. This masculine identification added to her existing tendencies toward bisexuality that was later reflected in her close idealizing relationship with Maria Lewis, a teacher at the boarding school.

The mother died in her early fifties when George Eliot was just 16. The effects of this traumatic loss during midadolescence, coupled with the earlier traumatic deprivation of a loving and responsive mother from infancy onwards, is striking evidence of severe traumatic scarring of her personality. She wrote in her journal in 1861, "What moments of despair that life would ever be made precious to me by the consciousness that I lived to some good purpose! It was that sort of despair that sucked away the sap of half the hours which might have been filled by energetic youthful activity . . ." (p. 254). This assessment of herself and her internal perception of an arrest is indicative of a deep insight into her inner life and her writing problem. She was not just superficially inhibited, though, since she was hampered by an inner turmoil that came to be represented particularly in a variety of symptoms indicative of a neurotic process: hypochondriacal preoccupations, migraines, and as a child night terrors. She was repeatedly sick with colds, was colicky, and had fears of Hell and Satan, an offended Deity, ghosts, etc. For a while, she turned to fundamentalist religion (Evangelicalism) after her idolized and idealized brother Isaac had grown up, married, and detached himself from the family.

Her mother's rejection and inability to function as a soothing, comforting shield, and her later death, the father's harsh rigid religiosity; and the brother's "abandonment" left deep scars that did not heal until she had thoroughly merged with Lewes. Only then did her depression fade enough for her to be able to make use of her extraordinary literary gift. Lewes actively encouraged her by constantly giving her the support she needed. Frightened by what success would bring her in terms of public recognition, he acted as a protective buffer between her and her curious, critical, but admiring public, as well as her capriciously picky publishers. He fulfilled the functions of husband-paternal-protector-encourager, but perhaps most importantly, the mirroring maternal function she had been so completely deprived of in childhood and adolescence. Her personality blossomed and flourished as so many analysands frequently do when they have experienced the favorable analytic container environment. Likewise, the interpretative work of the analytic situation produces the most precious gift of total, uncompromising understanding and activates or catalyzes creative new personality growth.

In adolescence, she became a voracious reader, after a slow educational start. At the Misses Franklin boarding school, she was a reasonably good student but not anything outstanding. Following her formal education, she had no choice but to return home to live with her strict, rigidly conservative father. Her capacities for independent thinking, however, briefly surfaced when she broke with her father's strict religious beliefs and refused to attend church services with him. He responded by shutting her out and giving her the cold shoulder. The fact that she had no occupation with which to support herself, her fears about separation, and her deep guilt-ridden sense of obligation, forced her to remain for some years with her father, and even nurse him in his final illness. She received neither moral nor emotional support from her older siblings who left it up to her to take care of the father. Later, though, without rancor she would generously send money to her sister when she needed it. But, for the time being, she was forced to reconcile with her father and though she outwardly resumed attendance at church services with him, she privately preserved her hard-won intellectual independence.

Serendipitously, they moved to a small cottage near Canterbury where fate delivered to her a nearby family of free thinkers, the Brays and Sara and Charles Hennel, who were at the center of a sophisticated rural group of liberal minded men and women. They welcomed her as a regular visitor and active participant in their discussions. As a result of her strict religious upbringing, however, she regretted to her dying days the pain she had caused her father. She wrote that genuine tolerance can occur only when the tolerant one can keep back his own views, not out of hypocrisy or superiority, but with a genuine desire to enter into the underlying feelings and views of another person. This was an early premonitory sign of her budding genius, according to Redinger, of the "gradual development of empathy that grew out of a selflessness, a strong conscience, and a freedom for self assertiveness to express her views unequivocally. Servants even came to her to reveal their innermost secret troubles. This development of her capacities for what she called 'tolerance' and Browning called 'burning power of sympathy' " (p. 127) is clearly what psychoanalysts now recognize as empathic understanding of the conscious and unconscious feeling states in another person. During the years before she met Lewes she was practicing those skills that would serve her well later on in her creation of believable, three-dimensional emotional characters in her novels.

She also began to immerse herself in various literary tasks such as the translation of Spinoza, Rousseau, and Strauss's *Life of Jesus*. At the same time, she got serially involved in a passionate idealization of a married man of the cloth and subsequently an impecunious art restorer. Strauss's views were rather painful to her since he was intent on demythologizing Jesus regarding Jesus' miracles as fabrications of His followers and the Apostles. Her work on Rousseau's *Confessions* augmented yet another facet of her talents, her capacities for self-observation, introspection, and analysis of what she perceived internally. Insightful conclusions followed to further enhance her novel writing. It is interesting to note that she counted as one of her closest friends in England, the famous Jewish intellectual Emmanuel Deutsch (Alexander, 1991) who was the inspiration for the character Mordecai in her novel *Daniel Deronda*. Mordecai's Jewishness and the psychological stresses of being adopted combined to produce the circumstances of a young man in search of his identity and self-esteem. Eliot focuses on his family romance fantasies as he develops from childhood into adolescence and into adulthood (Warner, 1993).

It was at this point, though, that her father died. Deep in her grief, she traveled to the Continent with the Brays, ending up in Switzerland where she stayed on for several months in Geneva. She met and lived with a family named the D'Alberts. M. D'Albert was a four-foot tall deformed painter who in time did a portrait of her, while Mme. D'Albert loved her and kissed her like a baby. George Eliot, in her regressed grief, called her "Maman." It is entirely possible she had an affair with M. D'Albert who then accompanied her back to England when she left Switzerland rather precipitously.

She must have recovered enough from her grief and low self-esteem to seek out the publisher of the *Westminster Review*, John Chapman, and ask for an editorial job. The *Westminster Review* had been a prestigious publication for some time since it was originally founded by John Stuart Mill's father and was headed by J. S. Mill for a time. But the *Review* had fallen on bad times and Chapman was energetically striving to revive it.

Here begins a very strange but fascinating chapter in George Eliot's life. She moved into the front room of the Chapmans' house on the Strand. She and Chapman were very much involved with each other and they entered into deep intellectual and literary discussions day and night. It is possible they had an affair, even though he already had a wife and a mistress who was the children's governess, both of whom joined together in jealously opposing the relationship between Eliot and Chapman. George Eliot solemnly promised to help him become what he wanted to be. This relationship was clearly very important to her intellectual and creative development as a writer. But it served another purpose as well since he was more like a transitional object in her consolidation of a sturdy self. She became the editor of the *Westminster Review* from 1851 to 1860 and saw to it that it was restored to its former high literary status. As time went on, though, she struggled to free herself from what had become a stifling relationship with Chapman who more openly demanded that she be his "second self" (p. 182). She fought with him and eventually moved out of the Chapman house in October 1853, but not without having someone waiting in the wings. In fact, she had met another young man by the name of Spencer who was the music critic for a London paper. Again, she engaged in a most intense relationship, spending many hours talking with him about literary subjects, music, philosophy, and religion. She accompanied him to many concerts. All these relationships (Isaac, Maria Lewis, the Brays, Sarah Hennel, the D'Alberts, Chapman, and Spencer) it seems to me were predominately transitional or idealized self-selfobjects with whom she entered into a merger that facilitated her personality development. But the most significant development was yet to come.

Late in the fall of 1853, when she was 32, she began an alliance with a man she had met two years before, George Henry Lewes, who was 34. He was "a versatile journalist, literary and drama critic, author of the astonishingly influential book *The Biographical History of Philosophy*, novelist, and adapter of foreign plays to the English stage" (Redinger, 1975, p. 227). He was a regular contributor to *The Leader*, a liberal weekly. Delightfully stimulating as a companion, an excellent conversationalist, and intellectually brilliant, he had a coruscating mind. Unfortunately and blindly, he had married a beautiful red-haired young woman who couldn't remain faithful and she gave birth to several children by Thorton Leigh Hunt, son of the famous literary critic Leigh Hunt. Amazingly and admirably, Lewes weathered this public humiliation even to the extent of supporting these children who, according to the laws at that time, took his name.

Earlier, Lewes had arrived in London as a young man and soon thereafter attached himself to Leigh Hunt, who incidentally was in the same literary circle with such luminaries as John Stuart Mill, Thomas Carlyle, and William Bell Scott. Lewes is described by Redinger as a strange looking, short, thin man with long wiry hair, full of fire and gesticulating enthusiasm about literature and drama. Elliot and Lewes were a perfect match, these two "outcasts." Both had loved before, and had been gravely disappointed and disillusioned in prior love relationships.

Redinger's accurate description of Eliot's personality consolidation process was of a slow gradual emergence as "a result of the subtly continuing modulating force of her writing present upon her buried past" (p. 5), a process familiar to clinical psychoanalytic work. Furthermore, just as the unconscious past is important in an analysis, George Eliot herself referred to her "primal passionate store" of past history that she drew on extensively and that it had "always been a vague dream" (p.

4) of hers to become a novelist. Jokingly, but tellingly and insightfully, George Henry Lewes wrote to Barbara Bodichon: "But, dear Barbara, you must not call her Marian Evans again: that individual is extinct, rolled up, mashed, absorbed in the Lewesian magnificance!" (p. 11). Similarly, her second husband John W. Cross, in his biography of her life, observed that "she showed from the earliest years, that trait that was most marked in her all through life, namely, the *absoluteness* of someone person who should be all in all to her and to whom she should be all in all" (p. 39).

In 1854, after translating Feuerbach's *The Essence of Christianity*, George Eliot wrote that "the free bond of love; for a marriage the bond of which is merely an external restriction, not the voluntary, contented self constriction of love, in short, a marriage which is not spontaneously willed, self sufficing, is not a true marriage" (p. 263). She then described her relationship with Lewes in an intellectual idiom: "the intense happiness of our union is derived in a high degree from the perfect freedom which we follow and declare our impressions" (p. 265). At the same time, Lewes wrote about Goethe's lack of a relationship with Fredericka that paralleled his contrasting relationship with George Eliot: "the exquisite companionship of two souls striving in emulous spirit of loving rivalry to become better, to become wiser, teaching the other to soar" (p. 265).

They left for the continent on July 20, 1854, and a month later, she put to paper her state of mind: "I am happier every day and find my domesticity more and more delightful and beneficial to me. Affection, respect, and intellectual sympathy deepens, and for the *first time* [emphasis added] in my life I can say to the moments 'verwielen sie, sie sind so schon' " (p. 267) (quotation from Faust). They stayed in Germany a couple of years, and the first thing she wrote was very similar in concept and content to what Lewes wrote about (as noted by Mathilde

Blind) the life of Goethe, monies from the publication of which supported them. She was working at that time on translating Spinoza's *Ethics*, which she completed in February 1856. Negotiations for the publication of this work broke down temporarily between Lewes and his publisher over some misunderstanding, which was unfortunate because she was worried over their desperate financial situation. It was in the context of their financial need that she initially began to write fiction for the first time, and *Scenes from a Clerical Life* was completed fifteen months later. Being emotionally supported and encouraged by Lewes was most important to her, but Lewes was constructively critical of her dramatic power, tactfully protective of her talents, and in exchange he borrowed her descriptive power. Their relationship was "comradely, sharing of interests, joys, and tribulations" (Redinger, 1975, p. 300). She was supportive of him, too, since she went with him later on to the Welsh coast to collect and study mollusks, zoophytes, annelids, and other sea creatures. Apparently, he was bent on writing a scientific essay on these animals to rebut Huxley's criticism that he was merely a book scientist.

In 1858 *Adam Bede* was completed and the following year she was hard at work on *The Mill on the Floss*. She was now three years into fiction writing. Redinger described the strange but intriguing sense of the creative act:

> It had taken three years of fiction writing for the full impact of the creative force to reach her and release memory from the practical duty of ordinary recall. It could then plunge downward in its relentless search for origins and set in motion the tantalizing dialectic of artistic creation—the need to find, to defend, but also to disguise the house of self that is buried under layers of time and feeling [p. 297].

Redinger gave three components to the creative act—confession, sympathy, and memory. *The Mill on the Floss* was written when she finally broke with her brother Isaac and consolidated her relationship with Lewes. It was her brother's constant disapproval of her lifestyle and his failure to communicate with her, even when he had deduced that she was the author of *Scenes from a Clerical Life* in which were descriptions of events no one else could have known about but Isaac and herself. It was from this point onwards that George Eliot's creativity flowered and flourished in the context of her relationship with Lewes.

SUMMARY

There are innumerable ways of conceptualizing creativity. for example, a neurobiological approach includes special cognitive skills; language and visual–spatial skills; an intense emotionality; a felicitous fitting in with a specific domain; investigating the unconscious motivations; intuition; fantasy life; timelessness; and just plain luck. The thesis, though, in this chapter is that the creative individual makes novel use of special gifts, talents, and the creative capacities to grow, transform narcissistic configurations and investments that are similar to the archaic transferences occurring in the analysis of narcissistic personalities. The gifted person discovers and realizes his or her creative potential during the expanding consolidating developmental period from late adolescence on into young adulthood. In addition, and most particularly, this personality consolidation is coupled with an intense interpersonal and intrapsychic relationship with a significant person that facilitates and "crystallizes" the surprisingly novel and creative original way of visualizing a particular piece of reality. Jack Stillinger's research (1991) suggests a similar conclusion from his studies of Keats' collaboration with his editors and friends.

It seems, then, that a close relationship with another person is at least one of the critically necessary elements in the production of great work whether it be literary, pictorial, or scientific, even in those individuals who have considerable difficulty forming relationships such as Turner and Newton. Winnicott's (1951) ideas of transitional objects are relevant here (see also Modele, 1970). Moreover, the September 24, 1994, to January 8, 1995, exhibition of the "Origins of Impressionism"at the Metropolitan Museum of Art in New York graphically pointed out the close collaboration of the Impressionist painters Manet, Monet, Brazille, and H. Fantin-Latour with each other and Emile Zola, the writer.

An interesting and most important question is how does psychoanalysis facilitate the recovery of the creative process when it has been derailed, or for that matter never released from some form of psychological paralysis and bondage. The thesis presented here suggests that when the developmental process has been set back on track through analysis of paralyzing conflicts and identity crises, creativity can reemerge and flower.

However, in those instances of psychopathological breakdown during this developmental period, such disorganizing disturbances can be seen to be derived from severe early childhood trauma that had led to serious, scarring defects in self organization, such as Conrad (Meyer, 1964d) and Woolf (Abse, 1994). These deficits in the organization of the self may leave an artist vulnerable to the "slings and arrows of outrageous fortune" (*Hamlet*, 1. line 58). These persons are unable to sustain creative experiences in the face of regressive pressures of overwhelming affects. Creativity in such instances gives rise to the frequent references in the literature (Lagercrantz, 1984; Lidz, 1964; Rothenberg, 1990; Ostwald, 1993) to the closeness between madness and creativity (e.g., Strindberg, Van Gogh, Robert Schumann, or Conrad) and creative work may continue sporadically or in a more chaotic or disorganized form. I agree with Noy (1979) that the neurotic or psychotic process is basically and intrinsically different from the creative process, although some researchers contend that the creative process is an attempt to heal a disorganized and fragmented self. Moreover, some severely brain damaged persons (excluding the *idiot savants* who exhibit an extraordinary isolated talent, but do not make original contributions) and alexithymic patients are less likely to be creative at all (Krystal, 1988). The young adult creative personality undergoes consolidation simultaneously with the presence of the synthetic function of a strengthened flexible ego that resists regression or in other terms is comprised of an emerging cohesive self.

Gruber's (1982) evolving systems approach to the study of creative individuals' lives is a fruitful way of discovering how total immersion and concentration of energies and skills within a specific domain tend to deliver a continuous series of connected and related creative contributions. George Eliot's life has been considered to show that for a person to be creative consolidation of the personality in young adulthood and a close personal relationship are critically necessary, in conjunction with a vivid imagination while maintaining a childlike freshness in enlivening a piece of reality along with the drive to create. Some psychoanalytic conceptualizations are offered to round out an understanding of creativity in the young adult.

REFERENCES

Abrams, M. H. (1987), Foreword. In: *William Wordsworth and the Age of Romanticism,* ed. J. Wordsworth, M. C. Jaye, & R. Woof with the assistance of P. Funnell. New Brunswick, NJ: Rutgers University Press.
Abse, D. W. (1994), Virginia Woolf: The urge to write. *Mind & Human Interact.,* 5:22–33.
Alexander, E. (1991), George Eliot's Rabbi. *Commentary,* 92:28–31.
Anderson, H. H. (1965), *Creativity in Childhood and Adolescence.* Palo Alto, CA: Science and Behavior.
Anderson, J. W. (1980), The process of creativity in the light of James's experience. In: *William James's Depressive Period (1867–1872) and the Origins of His Creativity: A Psychobiographical Study.* Doctoral dissertation, University of Chicago, Department of Behavioral Sciences, Committee on Human Development.

Armstrong, R. M. (1971), Joseph Conrad: The conflict of command. *The Psychoanalytic Study of the* Child, 26: 485–534. Chicago: Quadrangle.

Arnheim, R. (1976), The aesthetic approach: Notes on creativity. In: *Essays in Creativity,* ed. S. Rosner & L. E. Abt. Croton-on-Hudson, NY: North River Press, pp. 7–21.

Barth, J. R. (1977), *The Symbolic Imagination: Coleridge and the Romantic Tradition.* Princeton, NJ: Princeton University Press.

Barzun, J. (1989), The paradoxes of creativity. *Amer. Scholar,* 58:337–351.

Blos, P. (1962), *On Adolescence.* Glencoe, IL: Free Press.

Boorstin, D. J. (1992), *The Creators.* New York: Random House.

Brenman-Gibson, M. (1976), Notes on the study of the creative process. *Psychoanal. Inqu.,* 36:326–357.

Brettell, R., Cachin, F., Freches-Thory, C., & Stuckey, C., with Zegers, P. (1988), *The Art of Paul Gaugin.* Chicago: Art Institute of Chicago; Washington, DC: National Gallery of Art.

Bruner, J. (1968), *On Knowing.* New York: Atheneum.

Catalogue. The Wordsworth Project, Rutgers University-Newark, Department of English. Brochure prepared in conjunction with New York Council for the Humanities. Exhibition, New York Public Library, October 31–January 2, 1988.

Commons, M. L., Richards, F. A., & Armon, C. (1984), *Beyond Formal Operations.* New York: Praeger.

De Bono, E. (1969), *The Mechanism of Mind.* New York: Penguin.

Eissler, K. R. (1971), *Talent and Genius.* New York: Quadrangle Books.

—— (1978), Creativity in adolescence. *The Psychoanalytic Study of the Child,* 33:461–517. New Haven, CT: Yale University Press.

Erikson, E. (1958), *Young Man Luther.* New York: W. W. Norton.

—— (1969), *Gandhi's Truth.* New York: W. W. Norton.

Feldman, D. H. (1971), Map understanding as a possible crystallizer of cognitive structures. *Amer. Ed. Res. J.,* 8:485–501.

—— (1974), Universal to unique: A developmental approach to creativity. In: *Essays in Creativity,* ed. S. Rosner & L. E. Abt. Croton-on-Hudson, NY: North River Press, pp. 47–85.

—— (1982), A developmental framework for research with gifted children. In: *Developmental Approaches to Giftedness and Creativity.* San Francisco, CA: Jossey-Bass, pp. 31–45.

—— (1986), *Nature's Gambit.* New York: Basic Books.

—— (1991), Mozart as prodigy, Mozart as artifact. In: *The Pleasures and Perils of Genius: Mostly Mozart,* ed. P. Ostwald & L. S. Zegans. Madison, CT: International Universities Press, pp. 29–47.

Findlay, A. (1937), *A Hundred Years of Chemistry.* New York: Macmillan.

Fossi, G. (1985), Psychoanalytic theory and the problem of creativity. *Internat. J. Psycho-Anal.,* 66:215–230.

Freud, A. (1981), Insight: Its presence and absence as a factor in normal development. In: *The Psychoanalytic Study of the Child*, 36:241–249. New Haven, CT: Yale University Press.

Freud, S. (1907), Delusions and Dreams in Jensen's *Gradiva*. *Standard Edition*, 9:1–93. London: Hogarth Press, 1959.

——— (1908), Creative writers and day-dreaming. *Standard Edition*, 9:141–153. London: Hogarth Press, 1959.

Gardner, H. (1982), Giftedness: Speculations from a biological perspective. In: *Developmental Approaches to Giftedness and Creativity*, ed. D. H. Feldman. San Francisco, CA: Jossey-Bass, pp. 47–64.

——— Wolf, C. (1988), The fruits of asynchrony: A psychological examination of creativity. *Adol. Psychiatry*, 15:96–120. Chicago: University of Chicago Press.

Gay, P. (1988), *Freud: A Life for Our Times*. New York: W. W. Norton.

Gedo, J. E. (1988), Portrait of the artist as adolescent prodigy: Mozart and the Magic Flute. In: *Adol. Psychiatry*, 15:288–299. Chicago: University of Chicago Press.

——— (1994), The inner world of Paul Gaugin. *Annual of Psychoanalysis*, 22:61–109. Hillsdale, NJ: Analytic Press.

Gedo, M. (1980), *Art as Autobiography*. Chicago: University of Chicago Press.

Ghiselin, B. (1952), *The Creative Process*. New York: Mentor.

Gombrich, E. H. (1961), *Art and Illusion*, rev. ed. Princeton, NJ: Princeton University Press.

——— Hochberg, J., & Black, M. (1970), *Art, Perception, and Reality*. Baltimore: Johns Hopkins University Press.

Greenacre, P. (1959), Play in creative imagination. *The Psychoanalytic Study of the Child*, 14:61–80. New York: International Universities Press.

——— (1971), *Emotional Growth. Psychoanalytic Studies of the Gifted and a Great Variety of Other Individuals*, Vols. 1 & 2. New York: International Universities Press.

Grinstein, A. (1995), *The Remarkable Beatrix Potter*. Madison, CT: International Universities Press.

Gruber, H. E. (1982), On the hypothesized relation between giftedness and creativity. In: *Developmental Approaches to Giftedness and Creativity*, ed. D. H. Feldman. San Francisco, CA: Jossey-Bass.

——— (1989), The evolving systems approach to creative work. In: *Creative People at Work* ed. D. B. Wallace, & H. E. Gruber. New York: Oxford University Press, pp. 3–24.

Hamilton, J. W. (1975), Depersonalization in the life and writings of Joseph Conrad. *Psychoanal. Quart.*, 44:612–630.

——— (1979), Doppelganger effect: Joseph Conrad and Bertrand Russell. *Internat. Rev. Psychoanal.*, 6:175–182.

Hershman, D. J., & Lieb, J. (1988), *The Key to Genius*. Buffalo, NY: Prometheus Books.

Himmelfarb, G. (1994), George Eliot for grown-ups. *Amer. Scholar,* 63:577–581.

Hobbs, A. S., Whalley, J. I., & Taylor, J. (1987), The little books. In: *Beatrix Potter 1866–1943, The Artist and Her World.* London: Penguin, pp. 107–168.

Huscher, P. (1995), *Chicago Symphony Program Notes.* October 19, 20, 21 & 24.

James, W. (1890), *The Principles of Psychology,* Vol. 1. New York: Dover, 1950.

Japp, F. R. (1898), Kekule Memorial Lecture. *J. Chem. Soc.,* 73:97–138.

Jeffrey, L. R. (1989),Writing and rewriting poetry: William Wordsworth. In: *Creative People at Work,* ed. D. B. Wallace, & H. E. Gruber. New York: Oxford University Press, pp. 69–89.

Jones, E. (1953), *The Life and Work of Sigmund Freud,* Vol. 1. New York: Basic Books.

——— (1955), *The Life and Work of Sigmund Freud,* Vol. 2. New York: Basic Books.

——— (1956), The nature of genius. *Brit. Med. J.,* 2:257–262.

——— (1957), *The Life and Work of Sigmund Freud,* Vol. 3. New York: Basic Books.

Joseph, E. D. (1963), Identity and Joseph Conrad. *Psychoanal. Quart.,* 32:549–572.

Joyce, J. (1916), *A Portrait of the Artist as a Young Man.* New York: Modern Library.

Keats, J. (1958), *The Letters of John Keats,* ed. H. E. Rollins. Cambridge, MA: Harvard University Press, pp. 191–194.

Keegan, R. T. (1989), How Charles Darwin became a psychologist. In: *Creative People at Work,* ed. D. B. Wallace & H. E. Gruber. New York: Oxford University Press, pp. 107–125.

Kekule, A. (1865), Lecture. *Bull. Soc. Chim.,* 3:98–110.

——— (1866), Annalen. 137:129–130.

Keynes, J. M. (1956), Newton, the man. In: *The World of Mathematics,* ed. J. R. Newman. New York: Simon & Schuster, pp. 122–285.

Kligerman, C. (1957), A psychoanalytic study of the confessions of St. Augustine. *J. Amer. Psychoanal. Assn.,* 5:469–484.

Koestler, A. (1964), *The Act of Creation.* New York: Macmillan.

Kohut, H. (1959), Introspection, empathy, and psychoanalysis. *J. Amer. Psychoanal. Assn.,* 7:459–483.

——— (1966), Forms and transformations of narcissism. In: *Self Psychology and the Humanities. Reflections on a New Psychoanalytic Approach,* ed. C. B. Strozier. New York: W. W. Norton.

——— (1976), Creativeness, charisma, group psychology. Reflections on the self-analysis of Freud. In: *Self Psychology and the Humanities. Reflections on a New Psychoanalytic Approach,* ed. C. B. Strozier. New York: W. W. Norton.

Kris, E. (1952), *Psychoanalytic Explorations in Art*. New York: International Universities Press.

Krystal, H. (1988), On some roots of creativity. *Psychiatric Clin.*, 11:475–491.

Kubie, L. S. (1958), *Neurotic Distortion of the Creative Process*. Porter Lecture Series 22. Lawrence, KA: University of Kansas Press.

———— (1967), Blocks to creativity. In: *Explorations in Creativity*, ed. R. L. Mooney & T. A. Razik. New York: Harper & Row, pp. 33–42.

Lagercrantz, O. (1984), *August Strindberg*, tr. A. Hollo. New York: Farrar, Straus, Giroux.

Lane, M. (1946), *The Tale of Beatrix Potter*. New York: Penguin Books.

Leavey, S. A. (1970), John Keats's psychology of creative imagination. *Psychoanal. Quart.*, 39:173–197.

Lidz, T. (1964), August Strindberg: A study of the relationship between his creativity and schizophrenia. *Internat. J. Psycho-Anal.*, 45:399–418.

Liebert, R. S. (1983), *Michelangelo: A Psychoanalytic Study of His Life and Images*. New Haven, CT: Yale University Press.

Lindsay, J. (1973), *Turner, His Life and Work*. St. Albans, Herts: Panther Books.

Lowell, A. (1952), The process of making poetry. In: *The Creative Process*, ed. B. Ghiselin. New York: Mentor, pp. 109–112.

Lubin, A. J. (1977), From Augustine to Einstein. *Dialogue*. San Francisco: The Friends of the San Francisco Institute.

Mahon, E. J. (1987), Ancient Mariner, pilot's boy. A note on the creativity of Samuel Taylor Coleridge. *The Psychoanalytic Study of the Child*, 42:489–509. New Haven, CT: Yale University Press.

Mednick, S. A. (1962), The associative basis of the creative process. *Psychol. Rev.*, 69:220–232.

Meissner, W. W. (1994), Vincent van Gogh as artist: A psychoanalytic reflection. *Annual of Psychoanalysis*, 22:111–141. Hillside, NJ: Analytic Press.

Meyer, B. C. (1964a), Psychoanalytic studies on Joseph Conrad. I. The family romance. *J. Amer. Psychoanal. Assn.*, 12:32–58.

———— (1964b), Psychoanalytic studies on Joseph Conrad. II. Fetishism. *J. Amer. Psychoanal. Assn.*, 12:357–391.

———— (1964c), Psychoanalytic studies on Joseph Conrad. III. Aspects of orality. *J. Amer. Psychoanal. Assn.*, 12:562–586.

———— (1964d), Psychoanalytic studies on Joseph Conrad. IV. The ebb and flow of artistry. *J. Amer. Psychoanal. Assn.*, 12:802–825.

Mill, J. S., & Mill, H. T. (1970), *Essays on Sex Equality*, ed. A. S. Rossi. Chicago: University of Chicago Press.

Miller, A. I. (1989), Imagery and intuition in creative thinking: Albert Einstein's invention of the special theory of relativity. In: *Creative People at Work*, ed. D. B. Wallace & H. E. Gruber. New York: Oxford University Press, pp. 171–187.

Modell, A. (1970), The transitional object and the creative act. *Psychoanal. Quart.*, 39:240–250.

Muslin, H. (1995a), Ghandi. Unpublished typescript.
—— (1995b), Hitler. Unpublished typescript.
——Jobe, T. (1991), *Lyndon Johnson: The Tragic Self,* Psychoanalytic Portrait. New York: Plenum.
Nass, M. L. (1984), Development of creative imagination in composers. *Internat. Rev. Psychoanal.,* 11:481–492.
Newman, J. R. (1956), *The World of Mathematics.* New York: Simon & Schuster.
Noy, P. (1968), A theory of art and aesthetic experience. *Psychoanal. Rev.,* 55:623–645.
—— (1969), A revision of the psychoanalytic theory of the primary process. *Internat. J. Psycho-Anal.,* 56:155–178.
—— (1978), Insight and creativity. *J. Amer. Psychonal. Assn.,* 26:717–748.
—— (1979), Form creation in art: An ego psychological approach to creativity. *Psychoanal. Quart.,* 48:229–256.
—— (1985), Originality and creativity. *Annual of Psychoanalysis,* 12:421–448. New York: International Universities Press.
Ostwald, P. (1993), Genius, madness, and health: Examples from psychobiography. In: *The Pleasures and Perils of Genius: Mostly Mozart,* ed. P. Ostwald & L. S. Zegans. Madison, CT: International Universities Press, pp. 167–190.
—— Zegans, L. S., Eds. (1993), *The Pleasures and Perils of Genius: Mostly Mozart.* Madison, CT: International Universities Press.
Palombo, S. (1992), The eros of dreaming. *Internat. J. Psycho-Anal.,* 73:637–646.
Panel (1959), The psychology of imagination. Reporter: H. Kohut. *J. Amer. Psychoanal. Assn.,* 8:159–166.
Papajohn, G. (1995), Economics as a contact sport. *Chicago Tribune Magazine,* December 10, pp. 20–26.
Person, E., Fonagy, P., & Figueira, S. A., Eds. (1995), *On Freud's "Creative Writing and Daydreaming."* New Haven, CT: Yale University Press.
Piaget, J., & Inhelder, B. (1967), *The Child's Conception of Space.* New York: W. W. Norton.
Pinsky, R. (1988), Romantic and modern landscapes. Paper presented at the Chicago Historical Society, May 1.
Polanyi, M. (1969), The creative imagination. In: *Toward a History of Knowledge,* ed. H. Grene. *Psychological Issues,* Monogr. 22. New York: International Universities Press, pp. 53–70.
Proust, M. (1981), *Remembrance of Things Past,* tr. C. K. S. Moncrieff & T. Kilmartin. New York: Random/Vintage, 1971. Originally published Paris: Editions Gallimard, 1954.
Rathunde, K., & Csikszentmihalyi, M. (1993), Undivided interest and the growth of talent: A longitudinal study of adolescents. *J. Youth & Adol.,* 22:385–405.
Redinger, R. (1975), *George Eliot: The Emergent Self.* New York: Knopf.

Reed, M. L., Ed. (1991), *The Thirteen-Book of William Wordsworth*, Vols. 1 & 2. Ithaca, NY: Cornell University Press.

Richardson, D. (1989), *Pilgrimage*, 4 vols. New York: Knopf.

Rising, C. (1994), Conrad and Kohut: The fortunate oedipal tale. *Psychoanal. Contemp. Thought*, 17:107–120.

Rose, P. (1984), *Parallel Lives. Five Victorian Marriages.* New York: Vintage.

Rothenberg, A. (1990), *Creativity and Madness.* Baltimore: Johns Hopkins University Press.

Segal, H. (1984), Joseph Conrad and the mid-life crisis. *Internat. Rev. Psychoanal.*, 11:3–10.

Shakespeare, W. *The Complete Works of William Shakespeare*, ed. W. A. Wright. New York: Garden City, 1936.

Smith, G. J. W., & Carlsson, I. M. (1990), The Creative Processs: A Functional Model Based on Empirical Studies from Early Childhood to Middle Age. *Psychological Issues*, Monogr. 57. Madison, CT.: International Universities Press.

Snyder, B. R., & Tessman, L. H. (1965), Creativity in gifted students and scientists. In: *Creativity in Childhood and Adolescence*, ed. H. H. Anderson. Palo Alto, CA: Science and Behavior Books, pp. 21–34.

Solomon, M. (1995), *Mozart.* New York: HarperCollins.

Spitz, E. H. (1985), *Art and Psyche.* New Haven, CT: Yale University Press.

St. Augustine. *The Confessions of St. Augustine*, tr. E. B. Peas. London: Collier-Macmillan, 1961.

Stein, M. I., & Heinze, S. J. (1960), *Creativity and the Individual: Summaries of Selected Literature in Psychology and Psychiatry.* Glencoe, IL: Free Press.

Sterba, R. F. (1965), Remarks on Joseph Conrad's *Heart of Darkness. J. Amer. Psychoanal. Assn.*, 13:570–583.

Sternberg, R. J., & Davidson, J. E. (1983), Insight in the gifted. *Ed. Psychologist*, 18:51–57.

Stillinger, J. (1991), *Multiple Authorship and the Myth of Solitary Genius.* New York: Oxford University Press.

Strindberg, A. (1913), *The Red Room: Scenes of Artistic and Literary Life*, tr. E. Sprigge. London: Everyman's Library.

Tannenbaum, A. J. (1986), Giftedness: A psychosocial approach. In: *Conceptions of Giftedness*, ed. R. J. Sternberg & J. E. Davidson. Cambridge, U.K.: Cambridge University Press, pp. 21–52.

Taylor, J. (1986), *Beatrix Potter. Artist, Story Teller, and Countrywoman.* London: Penguin & Frederick Warne.

——— (1987), The story of Beatrix Potter. In: *Beatrix Potter 1866–1943: The Artist and Her World*, ed. J. Taylor, J. I. Whalley, A. S. Hobbs, & E. M. Battrick. London: Penguin Books, pp. 9–34.

Tinterow, G., & Loyrette, H. (1994), *Origins of Impressionism.* New York: Metropolitan Museum of Art.

Tolchin, N. L. (1988), *Mourning, Gender, and Creativity in the Art of Herman Melville*. New Haven, CT: Yale University Press.

Tweney, R. D. (1989), Fields of enterprise: On Michael Faraday's thought. In: *Creative People at Work*, ed. D. B. Wallace & H. E. Gruber. New York: Oxford University Press, pp. 91–106.

Wallace, D. B. (1989), Stream of consciousness and reconstruction of self, Dorothy Richardson's *Pilgrimage*. In: *Creative People at Work,*. ed. D. B. Wallace & H. E. Gruber. New York: Oxford University Press, pp. 147–169.

———— Gruber, H. E., Eds. (1989), *Creative People at Work*. New York: Oxford University Press.

Walters, J., & Gardner, H. (1986), The crystallizing experience: Discovering an intellectual gift. In: *Conceptions of Giftedness*, ed. R. J. Sternberg & J. E. Davidson. Cambridge, U.K.: Cambridge University Press, pp. 306–331.

Warner, L L. (1993), Family romance fantasy resolution in George Eliot's *Daniel Deronda*. In: *The Psychoanalytic Study of the Child*, 48:379–397. New Haven, CT: Yale University Press.

Weisberg, P. S., & Springer, K. J. (1961), Environmental factors in creative function. In: *Explorations in Creativity*, ed. R. L. Mooney & T. A. Razik. New York: Harper & Row.

Westfall, R. S. (1981), The career of Isaac Newton. *Amer. Scholar,* 50:341–353.

Whalley, J. I., & Hobbs, A. S. (1987), Fantasy, rhymes, fairy tales and fables. In: *Beatrix Potter, 1866–1943*. Harmondsworth, UK: Penguin, pp. 49–70.

Winnicott, D. (1951), Transitional objects and transitional phenomena. In: *Collected Papers*. London: Tavistock, 1958, pp. 229–242.

Wordsworth, J., Ed. (1987), *William Wordsworth: An Illustrated Selection*. Grasmere, U.K.: The Wordsworth Trust.

Young-Bruehl, E. (1991), *Creative Characters*. New York: Routledge.

Chapter 9

Summary and Conclusions

The period of life called young adulthood is coterminal with the ending of adolescence and the age group under consideration ranges from 18 years to the early thirties. These young people are in college, graduate school, or already in the workforce. In my opinion, young adulthood is *the most exciting* of all phases of development, particularly so, when it is contrasted with the hormonal/ physiological and psychological changes that dominate the beginning of the adolescent and pubertal period. What is so exciting is the fact the personalities of young adult people are in flux and engaged in a dynamic process of psychological consolidation. Physical maturation has been completed. The monumental developmental tasks of integration, synthesis, and cohesion of multiple areas of the personality result in a strikingly observable "settling down" into a chosen career, searching for and finding a suitable partner with whom to achieve physical and emotional intimacy, mastery of the drives, fitting in with a social group identity, and the consequent establishment of clearly defined sexual and gender identities. Most young people learn to master and negotiate these tasks and successfully manipulate the external world more or less to their advantage. These psychological processes occur in the context of a complex physiological and bidirectional sociological milieu that Engel (1977) originally termed the biopsychosocial model of human behavioral interactions.

To appraise the depth and extent of these personality developments, the modern clinician must be armed with an extensive array of psychoanalytically informed tools. But before any evaluation of this period can be intelligently achieved, all prior developmental phase specific tasks must be thoroughly investigated. Also, it must be remembered people mature physically, develop psychologically, and relate socially at widely different rates. The "late-bloomers" are familiar to educators, parents, and friends alike as well as the precociously gifted ones who appear grown-up beyond their years. Youthful idealism that revolutionized American culture in the 1960s can be understood not only in terms of high energy levels, but also in terms of a significant restructuring of the superegos and ego ideals. Today's youth may not be as caught up in the same kind of revolutionary zeal, but they nevertheless undergo radical changes internally and exert an impact on society as a whole. There is a freeing up of narcissistic energies that provides easier access to creative talents in the arts and sciences. Perceptual and intellectual competencies are much freer of conflict so that intellectual study and formal operations are now more than ever possible for them to make significant contributions. In a word, the modern youth is transformed into at best a delightful, creative, intellectual, and seriously disciplined person. The educational environment promotes emotional, intellectual, and linguistic skills. From a sociological perspective, peers, professors, and siblings add a significantly rich menu of stimulation. In fact, young adults often report that certain professors and mentors were crucially important in their overall development, choice of a career, and a lifelong friendship so that young adults learn to cope and adapt to new circumstances. Cognitive development proceeds from lower levels of abstract thinking to postformal operations. Vygotsky's (1981) theories concerning the semiotic function of the educational environment and the use of language and symbolic thinking processes add significantly to the development of youth.

But it is the very nature of this transformation that makes the youthful person vulnerable to developmental failures in the transition from late adolescence into young adulthood. The felicitous and uncomplicated developmental trajectory may be derailed by combined internal and external pressures on the personality in transition. Sociological support systems normally shift from the values and standards of parents and extended family to new authority figures and peers, thus creating new and revised standards and values. This leaves the young adult in a moral and ethical vulnerable state. Premature involvement or failures in establishing sexual relationships can cause serious problems in establishing a lasting capacity for intimacy. Fragmentation and regression or arrested developmental processes then produce various psychopathological outcomes. Identity crises, identity diffusions, and various delays as originally defined by Erikson (1959, 1968) and elaborated by Marcia (1980) help the clinician to understand these problems of identity formation. For example, the Don Juan character, the person prone to narcissistic rage, and strivings for power are given flesh and sinew with in-depth psychoanalytic clinical material.

The Don Juan character is consumed with stereotypically persistent attempts to merge with an idealized mother based on an early childhood relationship with her that was characterized by overstimulation and sexualization. The person who strives for power also seeks a merger with the idealized mother, but unconsciously she is perceived as the invincible, grandiose, and omnipotent parent who will invariably relieve the child's distress of helplessness, loneliness, and fears of abandonment. Furthermore, she vicariously seeks power through her child. This explanation may fit the life story of some politicians. The philosophy of power was conceived by Nietzsche (1886) and Hobbes (1651) as a strong will and restless desire to dominate and control others that reminds one of Freud's aggressive drive and later his death instinct. Power is knowledge, money, rhetoric, athleticism, control of the media, and a system of higher values and morals. Military leaders display a denial of danger, believe themselves invincible, and take unusual risks to surprise the enemy in battle. Power struggles emerge in marriages, in corporate hierarchies, and in academia as well as in political movements and government. The analyst is perceived to exert power over his analysands by his expectant attention to unknown unconscious contents that are interpretable in the light of the psychoanalytic theory of repression and primary process thinking. Clinical material is presented to support the ideas about the use of power in the young adult.

Repeated and outrageous humiliations in childhood and adolescence very often lead to a narcissistic rage that has so violently erupted in schools recently. Homer's *Iliad* provides the opportunity to compare the clinical study of the internal processes of narcissistic rage with that of the literary and mythical character of Akhilleus whose mourning for his alter ego Patroklos led to the resolution of his rage. Disorders of sexual and gender identity are exaggerated during young adulthood. Sexual orientation issues for gay and lesbian young adults are especially poignant when they are "coming out," especially in terms of how to reveal their sexual orientation to family and friends. The social pressures to be "straight" for some are almost insurmountable. The call for well-designed longitudinal research is needed to obtain more accurate data about gay and lesbian youth than has been available through retrospective studies.

Creativity is the ultimate and most remarkable achievement in gifted individuals whose gifts are special and novel. In the young adult, two very important features come together in creative acts. One is the presence of a close personal relationship with a significant other and the other involves the processes of consolidation of the personality leading to freed up energies that can be devoted to creative endeavors. Anecdotal examples taken from literary and scientific discoveries are given, but the life of George Eliot is a thoroughly rich example of the thesis. Redinger's (1975) biography permits an in-depth study of the emergence of her talent as a first rate fiction writer of the nineteenth century. It interesting that it was within the context of the stimulation and support of her lifelong chosen partner George Henry Lewes that her talent came to life.

REFERENCES

Engel, G. L. (1977), The need for a new medical model: A challenge for biomedicine. *Amer. J. Psychiatry*, 137:535–544.

Erikson, E. H. (1959), Identity and the Life Cycle. *Psychological Issues*. Monogr. 1. New York: International Universities Press.

——— (1968), *Identity: Youth and Crisis*. New York: W. W. Norton.

Hobbes, T. (1651), *English Works, Vol. 7, Leviathan*. London: J. M. Dent, 1976.

Homer, (1920), *The Iliad of Homer*, ed. & tr. R. Lattimore. Chicago: University of Chicago Press.

Marcia, J. E. (1980), Identity in adolescence. In: *Handbook of Adolescent Psychology*, ed. J. Adelson. New York: John Wiley, pp. 159–187.

Nietzsche, F. (1886), *The Will to Power*, ed. W. Kaufmann & R. J. Hollindale. New York: Random House, 1967.

Redinger, R. (1975), *George Eliot: The Emergent Self*. New York: Knopf.

Vygotsky, L. S. (1981), The genesis of higher mental functions. In: *The Concept of Activity in Soviet Psychology*, ed. J. V. Wertsch. Armonk, NY: M. E. Sharpe.

Name Index

Abelin, E. L., 53, 75, 82
Abend, S. M., xxiii, 42–43
Abraham, K., 9
Abrams, M. H., 223
Abse, D. W., 213, 235, 247
Adams, G. R., 11, 40–41, 48
Adatto, C., 1, 16
Adler, A., 146
Ahamma, I. M., xx
Alexander, E., 241
Alexander, F., 4
Allison, A., xx
Altschul, S., 11
Anderson, H. H., 226
Anderson, J. W., 211, 212–213, 226
Appignanesi, L., 202
Appollonios of Rhodes, 190
Aristotle, 203
Arlin, P. A., xxiii
Arlow, J. A., 197, 202
Armon, C., 214
Armon, S., xxiii
Armstrong, R. M., 213
Arnaud, S. H., xxiv, 47
Arnheim, R., 231
Arnold, M., 201–202
Arnstein, R. L., 1
Aronfreed, J., 52
Arrow, C. N., 1, 19–20
Astin, A. W., xvi

Augustine, St., 221
Austen, J., 91, 124
Axelrod, S., 82

Balint, M., 52, 81
Balogh, T., 188
Barbier, J., 89–90
Barnett, M., 79
Barth, J. R., 227–228
Barzun, J., 217
Beautrais, A. L., xix
Beauvoir, S. de, 125
Bell, R. Q., 6
Benedek, T., 3, 16, 19, 75, 76, 80
Benson, E. F., 145n, 153–154, 211
Bergman, A., 18, 52, 81, 157
Bernays, J., 202
Bernstein, H., 38
Bettelheim, B., 71
Bibring, E., 195
Bibring, G., 25
Black, M., 215
Blackwell, T., 202, 203
Block, J., 1
Bloom, A., 47–48
Blos, P., 1, 4, 7, 18, 26, 157, 162, 218, 226
Blumstein, P., 173
Bondi, H., 62

Subject Index

273